LESS WINE
MORE TIME

MIM JENKINSON

ISBN: (sc) 978-0-6487637-0-3

general – non-fiction

Cover photography by Kate Sommer Photography

DEDICATION

To my husband, my babies and my closest family and friends who have always loved me, no matter what.

FOREWORD

We live in an age of authenticity and honesty. This means we understand the value that comes from being ourselves regardless of the occasion, and the value of speaking our truth to help others.

Authenticity and honesty tumble out of Mim like sand through an hourglass.

I have had the privilege of meeting and getting to know Mim through the AusMumpreneur Network, a nationwide community of mothers who are all building something special in business for themselves, and for their families.

What struck me from the first conversation with Mim was her natural warmth and rawness; I could immediately tell she was proud to be this version of herself. She's also the kind of person you can't help but gravitate towards - she'll open her heart to you without hesitation, make you laugh, and show a genuine interest in your story too.

As I have got to know Mim's personal story, I've realised – as you will too reading this book – that being who she is now – a strong, confident, goal-driven businesswoman - has not happened by accident. In the pages of this book, she shares with us stories throughout her life that led her to see alcohol as a solution to her challenges, rather than a slippery slope to a place where even she failed to recognise who she was anymore.

To read about her recognition that she had a problem, and the ways she turned her situation around to create a life she loves for herself and her family, is nothing short of inspirational. As a mum to two small children myself, running a successful business and writing books, I know all too well the temptation of that glass of wine once the house is still and it's time to finally sit and breathe. One glass can turn into three, every night, in the blink of an eye. It takes courage to understand that this situation is no longer an occasional occurrence; it's a proper addiction that can impact your life significantly, and that of those you love, if not addressed with urgency.

Like me, I know you'll devour the pages of this book and be thankful for the Mim's of this world – the ones not afraid to stand confidently in front of us and reveal their challenges, plus solutions to those challenges, to help others navigate the same, or similar circumstances.

Lisa Burling

Award-winning Businesswoman & Author

CONTENTS

Introduction   *1*

My Story   *7*

How I Got Addicted   *59*

The Turning Point   *66*

Breaking My Habit Day by Day   *77*

The Reaction from Family and Friends   *99*

Life After Alcohol   *111*

Motherhood and Alcohol - Why Do Mums Drink?   *122*

Strategies for Sobriety   *159*

What's Next for Me?   *175*

Summary   *179*

Resources

Acknowledgments

About the Author

INTRODUCTION

"It's ok, Mummy is just a bit car sick."

This is what my five-year-old daughter said to her three-year-old brother as we pulled up to the side of the road. So I could throw up the contents of my probable alcohol-poisoned stomach.

It was the first in a series of incidents that led me to the realisation I had a problem with alcohol.

Not a small problem. A big mother of a problem. One might call it alcohol addiction. I certainly would.

I have a story to tell you about how I slowly and steadily fell into the alcohol trap and how it ended up consuming my life.

How becoming a mother, and all that goes with the trials and tribulations of motherhood contributed to the addiction that consumed me.

It isn't a sad or sorry story filled with destruction and mortification. Well, there's a little of the latter. It's the story of an average mum of two, who, on the outside, had it all together, was in control, functioning and highly achieving. But behind closed doors was drinking heavily most nights. And could not stop.

Why? You'll soon find out.

This isn't a guidebook but a journey through my life over the past few years and the problems I've faced and overcome.

Never in a million years did I imagine one day I would quit alcohol. *Why would I?* Everyone drinks, don't they? And it's so much fun.

I didn't have a problem. And I didn't, until I did.

I never planned to quit. I just wanted to cut back. But I couldn't. Not even by one glass or one night a week by the end.

I'm going to assume you're a mother too and my story is already ringing a bell for you. You know, "mummy wine time."

Wine O'clock.

Mummy's special juice.

Mummy NEEDS wine.

And this is a judgement-free zone. I'm not here to shame you, call you out or tell you you're doing something wrong.

This is *my* story and I will share the issues I've faced and the steps I took to help myself.

When I say I'm better at something because I no longer drink, I'm talking about the person I am now versus the person I was before.

I won't gloss over the mess nor will I downplay the success either. I won't paint myself as a crumpled heap because my life is good, and I've already achieved a lot. But I was at the point where I suspect I might have lost it all.

I dreaded that one day a call would come to tell me my world had fallen apart because I could no longer control my consumption of alcohol. I've had that call in my life once before, when I was diagnosed with cancer. I strongly suspected I was heading for another one that might rip my family apart all over again.

It's the reason sharing this is so important to me. To see if this is happening in other mothers' lives too. To see if there is a growing dependency on alcohol to simply survive motherhood. Or so the social media memes would have you believe. We don't just *want* alcohol; we *need* it.

It was my secret.

The amount and frequency I was drinking, and the reasons for it, may shock you. But you know what shocks me the most? The fact no one knew I had a problem. Not even my nearest and dearest family and friends.

Since I've stopped drinking, my opinions about alcohol and why others drink has changed drastically. And it's oh-so-hard for me not to leap to judgement at times. But I'm trying to keep myself in check about that because who am I to say someone else has a problem?

When I've talked to people about why I stopped drinking, it's come with the caveat I'm talking about my personal experience.

I also reached out to my mum friends, my readers and my network of mothers to learn their opinions, habits and challenges about their own consumption of alcohol.

In fact, 1000 mothers provided insights when they answered my survey on Motherhood and Alcohol in May-June 2019. I share the results within this book and, let me say right now, it's eye-opening.

It amazed me how quickly these mothers voiced their opinion and experience of alcohol consumption since becoming a mum.

Has drinking high amounts of wine or gin become a rite of passage into fully functioning motherhood?

Has the media and entertainment industry created and perpetuated an increasingly high number of mothers with alcohol dependency? Or does a problem even exist?

I have my own opinions in answer to these questions and they're open to challenge. I'm not putting myself out here as an authority on mothers who drink but I want to lift a lid on the subject and start an open discussion about it.

The link between motherhood and alcohol.

Since the 18th century, we've often referred to gin as 'Mother's Ruin', according to The Cambridge Dictionary.

Source:https://dictionary.cambridge.org/dictionary/english/mother-s-ruin

Distilled in England in huge amounts and sold cheaply to the masses, it quickly became the vice and undoing of many mothers.

Even today, jokes, phrases and memes connecting 'mothers' and 'gin' are rife. If you don't drink gin, are you even a mother? *Have you heard that one, or similar?*

Why do so many mums become reliant on alcohol?

The survey results hold many answers to this.

And by answering my questions, respondents also shared hundreds of comments, trends and insights into their reasons for drinking alcohol and the portrayal of "mummy wine time" in the media.

It seems we don't all turn to drink for the same reasons but there are common trends that shocked me.

Back to me though.

If you've picked up this book to find out how I became addicted to alcohol, why it happened and what I did to undo the addiction, that's exactly what you'll get.

I understand how the prospect of quitting alcohol altogether seems drastic and unnecessary for some. I also get how terrifying it is when you're stuck in the alcohol trap and can't find a way out.

In this book, I will share the deepest, darkest secrets and situations I've hidden from so many for so long.

Embarrassment doesn't cover it but risking humiliation is worth it because sharing my personal experience with alcohol addiction has already helped so many.

So, expect real and raw. Expect honesty and anecdotes. But also, courage, substance and strength.

I'll tell you how I knew I had a real problem and the exact steps I took to fixing it.

I will share:

- How I became addicted to alcohol – from my first drink, aged six
- The turning point after realising I had a problem
- How I broke the habit of alcohol addiction and the first 100 days after becoming alcohol-free
- The surprising reactions from my closest family and friends
- The benefits I've discovered since becoming a non-drinker
- Insights into why other mothers drink alcohol and why some are susceptible to alcohol addiction

Since quitting, my life has changed dramatically for the better and continues to flourish. If only I had known how easy it would be for me.

For now, I'll tell you more about that side-of-the-road #badmum moment and all the embarrassing episodes that led to it.

MY STORY

At 9am on January 1st, 2019 I rolled over in bed at my best friend's house to reach over the bedside table to find a hangover-reducing, thirst-quenching glass of water.

The night before had been New Year's Eve, and it had been a big one. A day in the sun, drinking with friends, playing darts (I know, how 80s!) and slinging back the bubbles.

By midday, after eating all the carbs I could find in the house, I averted the crisis.

The headache left, copious amounts of water had rehydrated my parched body and brain and I was back in the land of the living. Which was a good thing given my kids were running around like maniacs and my husband needed a rest too.

But whilst millions of people around the globe were choosing New Year's Day as the start of their newfound sobriety, or at least 'cutting down the booze a bit', nothing was stopping me.

That day I paced myself, flitting between chatting, playing games and swimming with the kids and sunbathing. By 7pm, the kids were asleep, the socialising amped up, and the wine poured freely once more.

It's all a bit of a haze but I remember my glass never being empty and me never putting it down. I distinctly recall the occasional look of annoyance on my best friend's face and not knowing why it was there. Not really caring either—because I was having So. Much. Fun.

What was his problem?

The morning after, my comeback wasn't on par with the previous day. I practically fell out of bed at around midday, somehow showering before slinking downstairs to lie on the sofa, throwing myself an unglorified pity party for one.

My best friend, his fiancé and my husband didn't seem to suffer as much as I was. Whilst no one said anything, I had the most uncomfortable paranoia I'd done or said, something I shouldn't have done last night. I remember that annoyed look on my friend's face.

Eventually, we packed up, said our thank yous and piled into the car for the one-hour drive home.

Food. That's what I needed. Salty food and a shit tonne of water.

McDonalds was around the corner. Awesome. The perfect combo of grease, salt and fat would sort this out rapidly. Always does.

It didn't. I sat like a zombie in the front passenger seat of our car in McDonalds car park. My glazed eyes stared out the window as I attempted to chew a limp, salty fry before giving up altogether.

The drive home began and five minutes in I threw my hands up, frantically and wordlessly signalling to my husband to pull-the-hell-over.

Throwing open the car door, out came the contents of last night's booze binge into the grass. The hubs threw a towel over me and I attempted to clean myself up, but it kept coming. It hurt, it really hurt every inch of me.

When the episode was done, he returned to the driver's side and asked if it was ok to set off again. I nodded grimly.

"Are you ok, Mummy?" my three-year-old son, who had been sitting quietly in the back of the car, asked. Shit.

"Mummy is a bit car sick," my five-year-old daughter confidently confirmed, proud of her diagnosis.

"Yes," I replied, full of a deep shame my two babies had just witnessed me chucking up in such a dramatic fashion at the side of the road. "I feel better now. It's ok," I told them.

Of course, it was far from that.

Because at forty, this married mother of two was not ok. I was addicted to alcohol, and I didn't know how to stop.

In fact, I didn't want to stop. But I wanted to 'cut down'.

That's what people say isn't it? "I'm cutting down."

"I don't have a *problem*; I just need to cut down."

Well, I can't speak for them but cutting down wasn't an option for me. First, because I couldn't. I had tried for months to reduce the frequency and quantity I was drinking. I couldn't do it.

Second, well I've always been a bit of an 'all or nothing' kind of girl.

One glass of wine has never interested me.

As much as I might like to pretend I was drinking for the taste of wine, to gently relax after a hard day or to congratulate a friend on their wedding day. I wasn't.

I was drinking to get drunk. To escape, to forget, to be someone else. So many reasons I'll go into more in this book.

So 'cutting down' would never cut it for me.

But back to the kids. I'd longed to be a mother all my life and now had these two tiny humans depending on me for their own.

I'm a good mum.

I love my children and tell them often. I provide for them; I care for them; I ensure they have everything they need and every privilege I can afford them.

But after my drinking habit spiralled out of control, I would lie in bed at night, most nights, with a horrifying realisation. If something happened to one of them that night, I couldn't even drive them the ten-minute journey to the local hospital.

I'm a bad mum.

That's what I would tell myself. What a terrible mother you are, to put your own happiness before the safety of your children.

What if they needed me? Or something happened to my husband? What if he needed me?

And there I was, feeling like the world's worst out-of-control mother and wife and not capable of doing a single thing about it.

It was enough to make me want to drink. And it did. As did a bunch of other stuff.

Shall I let you know how it all started?

My first alcoholic drink - age six.

It's 1984 and at age six, I have my first alcoholic drink. Unless you include the brandy on my dummy, then it might have been more like six months.

Back in the 80s, kids over the age fourteen (I think) could legally drink at home. Or that's what they told us. I think that got blurred somewhat by my family as I was around six years old when I had my first taste of wine.

It was a tiny taste, offered by a family member who I love dearly.

To this day, we still laugh a lot about how after that first taste, I banged on the table and demanded, "More wine!"

I was six though and I cannot remember the event personally, but they've recounted the story so many times I can now vividly almost see and imagine every detail. Except the taste itself.

I can't imagine what six-year-old Mim thought of the taste of wine.

Would I have scrunched up my nose at the poison in front of me or would the sugar content have made it seem like a sweet treat?

I can picture myself taking it in, two small hands wrapped around a large glass of wine, excitedly taking a sip.

That's been me ever since actually, just with less of the banging and more inclination to get my own now.

My first alcohol-induced vomit - age fourteen.

It's 1992 and I'm invited on a night out to see a band with a friend, his older sister and her even-older boyfriend.

I'm sitting in a dark pub somewhere in Manchester, illegally clutching a bottle of Budweiser and feeling like the bees-fucking-knees.

I thought of myself as a bit of a rock chick—in my head.

So, this was bloody perfect.

I am cool. I'm so cool. Look at me being all cool in a bar, drinking beer out of the bottle and being cool.

I don't remember going to the bar myself, but I've always paid my way and assume I hand over my cash for more beers.

Getting home a few hours later was a blur but I have a hazy recollection of vomiting at the side of my bed. Not cool.

Something also 'not cool' was my mum discovering said vomit the next day because I'd forgotten I'd put it there and in my hungover stupor apparently couldn't smell it either. So gross.

Another story my family has dined out on for years.

There were some other occasions during my teenage years where I drank too much and barely remember what happened.

Such as the time I threw up noodles all over my friend's bathroom when her parents were out of town and she threw a party.

I denied that incident until I was blue in the face although I was the only partygoer who had ordered noodles from the Chinese takeaway. And I was *green* in the face the day after from too much alcohol.

The first time I vomited in a taxi - age eighteen.

It's 1997 and I'm eighteen years old.

I was working as a waitress in a cocktail bar.

No, no, I wasn't really. But I was working in the local pub in my first bartending job. This pub, well it was *the* pub to work at in my town.

I was working there practically every evening, loving the atmosphere and the oh-so-cool status I had decided working there ascribed me. It's now I realise how much approval I sought from others in my teen years. At the time, I would have told you I was the most confident one out of all my friends.

Some deep longing to be considered popular, cool and interesting has followed me all my life.

In the evenings working in the pub I got to know a local, Tony. I was eighteen; he was twenty-six. Now *that* was cool, right?

One night, we stayed behind after hours with the bar manager and another colleague. They poured drink after drink, and I kept up with my older peers, laughing, dancing and playing pool until midnight.

My new boyfriend bought me home safely in a taxi to where I was still living with my parents.

As we pulled up, the cab came to a stop, and I unceremoniously threw up on the floor of the car. Fuck.

I mean, five seconds later and it would have been on the pavement at least.

I don't remember anything after that but somehow must have dragged my sorry self up the steps, into the house and to bed.

At around midday the next day, I crawled out of bed after hearing my parents speaking with someone at the front door.

Couldn't they keep it down? I was tired!

"You have the wrong house!" they were firmly telling the man who stood outside. "My daughter has absolutely not been sick in your taxi!"

Oh, sweet Jesus, this is not happening.

And whilst they laughed a little in later years, I can imagine the deep humiliation they must have felt during that conversation with the poor taxi driver. And the deep disappointment they must have felt in me for behaving in such a way.

The first time I fell in love - age nineteen.

A year later, I met the man I thought I would marry. Like, for reals.

In a whirlwind few months, we'd moved in together and got engaged. Oh, and I'd had sex for the first time with him during a very drunken night.

Both were intentional, the drinking and the sex. At that age I was already learning alcohol blocked out pain. I knew with enough of it, I would be brave enough to do the deed and hopefully not feel a thing.

It wasn't the most romantic encounter, but a quick poll of my friends told me it wasn't for them the first time either.

However, I loved this boy and despite being so young; I thought I was one of the lucky ones. To have found true love so young and to be so happy and set up in our bubble together.

The bubble though, well, it got boring over time. Complacency set in quick and over the three years we were together, we changed from being 'love's young dream' to 'old before our time'. We stayed at home, ate junk food and drank cheap wine. A lot of it.

I suppose I lost interest in him and I started taking less

care of myself. Over the two years we were together, I piled on weight which led to me physically wanting to hide indoors. In our safe little home together, drinking bottles of wine. Gone was the fun-loving, sassy and adventurous girl he'd first met. I wasn't even pretending to be confident anymore. I wanted to go to work, come home and stay there.

But he was a twenty-two-year-old man with ambition and he eventually sussed the girl I'd become wasn't right for the journey he'd set himself on.

And on the day he told me he didn't love me anymore, he broke my already-fragile heart.

He said there wasn't anyone else involved, but he'd realised I was no longer right for him. I was boring; I didn't have any drive, and I didn't pay him enough attention. I had done badly wrong.

Of course, a few days later he came clean and told me he'd met someone else and was leaving me for her. *There's almost always someone else, isn't there?*

But the original reasons he'd given me were not wrong. I had stopped trying for myself, him and our life.

He had too though. I wonder if he ever realised that or still puts 100% of the blame on me.

We were both guilty of neglecting each other but whilst I stopped caring for myself too; he looked after himself well. He went to the gym, he found new friends, and he enjoyed nights out with the boys. He lived the life twenty-two-year-olds should be living.

He left me because he felt our relationship was boring and someone more exciting had caught his eye.

All that booze and I wasn't as interesting as I thought I

was.

During the separation period, he left his mobile phone in my car and I slyly listened to his voicemail. Replacement 'me' had left a slurred answerphone message for him with two words, "I'm drunk" before giggling and hanging up.

"What a desperate state!" I said out loud, as if I could judge.

I wondered if, when leaving that message, she might have thought herself cute or flirtatious, but she sounded as she was. Drunk.

I picked up my broken heart and took it back home to live with my parents and regroup with them.

When you're single as an adult, you learn what you'll do differently in the next relationship. What you'll do better, what changes you'll make and the behaviours you'll never tolerate again.

I was about to learn a lot.

My first time as a singleton - age twenty-two.

It's 2001 and I've moved into a girly pad in Manchester with my best friend, Niamh, to mend our broken hearts together. And to have as much fun as we could find.

See that big bee over there? We are the bee's knees. We really are.

We're living the life. We're not "Sex in the City", we're the Spice Girls. Complete with platform trainers and sass for days. We have actual Girl Power.

We rush through our workdays, then faff at the gym for thirty minutes and head out on the town. Oh yes, it's ladies' night, every night.

After the love and care of my parents, I was feeling back to my old self again; the strong, independent, passionate and ambitious woman I'd forgotten I was.

Being a single adult, as lonely as it might occasionally have got, was the making of me.

I mean, I wasn't a weak kitten before my last relationship, but I had become used to relying on my ex for a lot more than I needed to.

I enjoyed discovering new things, meeting new people, learning about the things I did and didn't like. I loved being brave, adventurous, and I also liked kissing boys. Lots of them. Fun times!

I lost weight, made more effort with my appearance and threw myself into my job at a global stockbroker and the social life that came with it.

Nights out in the local pub my colleagues pretty much owned were the feature of every other weeknight. And at the weekend, Niamh and I worked our way through the club scene in Manchester, relishing every second of our new single statuses.

She had been royally dumped at the same time as I was, and we pieced our broken hearts back together by snogging boys on sticky dance floors along with a few too many alcopops.

Niamh and I had a ball in our new city pad and the time we spent there rebuilt our confidence. Niamh's work colleagues dubbed us 'Muriel' and 'Stanley' because of the couple-like nature of our friendship. We did everything together; we finished each other's sentences, and we looked after each other. I was the Scary to her Ginger, the Posh to her Baby. To be fair, neither of us were particularly Sporty.

We also drank a fair bit of wine a little too frequently. It's what single girls do though, right? The telly says so.

After a night out, I threw up in a taxi again.

When I say, 'night out', I think it was about 8pm but I'd been drinking since mid-afternoon with the work crowd, on an empty stomach.

Niamh took me home and as we pulled up to the flat we were sharing, I chucked up right there in the cab.

Why, why?! That was another £15 not-so-well spent and another story to add to the Drunken Mim Chronicles.

Thing is, these stories didn't signify I had a problem with alcohol.

I mean, I was doing what every other teenager and young adult was doing, right? Learning their limits with alcohol, trying to blend in and be accepted by their peers. Throwing up in taxis.

My stories may horrify you or they might pale into insignificance when you recount your own drunken episodes.

The second time I fell in love - age twenty-two.

Over the years, drinking wine became an even more regular occurrence, and it was on a work night out that I met my next boyfriend.

At age twenty-two, at the office Christmas party, I met Damian and fell in love at first sight. We joked for years about the moment our eyes met, and we just 'knew'. We did, we just knew!

It was another whirlwind romance that saw me quit

my job and move to another city to be with him.

We bought our first home together after just two months. A tiny two-bed terraced house in Leeds that we dubbed the 'mini happy house'. And we were just that, blissfully happy.

This time, things were different.

Damian and I were best friends with benefits, spending half of our time having sex and the other half laughing until we cried.

We did everything together; we shared our circle of friends and were inseparable.

Our days out, nights in, holidays and happy adventures went on for another eighteen months when we moved into a new house together. A larger, three-bedroom home with a beautiful kitchen and endless space for entertaining friends.

Spoiler alert: this house was eventually named the 'big unhappy house', which was a shame.

Nothing was wrong in our relationship for a long time or nothing we could have put a finger on.

But one day, the realisation hit me we were probably not right for each other. I suppose as much as we loved every inch of each other, the real passion was gone.

Damian was still my best friend, but nothing more.

And I could see how easy it would have been to stay together, to get married and start a family. But likely, we would have cheated on each other.

On the outside, we were living a perfect life. We went out, we holidayed, we did home-renovations. We threw our own parties and went to parties together and we drank a lot.

The social life we had was heavily centred on drinking and it was another hobby we shared well together.

Our relationship would have continued to look perfect to outsiders. But as I mentioned earlier, I suspect we would have cheated on each other, even if we had never left each other. I didn't want that for us; I didn't want us to have an unhappy ending.

So, one day I asked for 'the talk' and confided all of this to him.

Telling your best friend, who you love to bits, that you don't think you want to be with him anymore without really knowing why, was crazy hard.

It was difficult to find the words and, having been so harshly cast aside myself years ago, I didn't want to inflict that pain on Damian.

He cried. And I cried.

We cried and hugged for about thirty minutes and at the end; we laughed. Laughed!

He felt the same as me, you see. We had both come to the realisation at the same time that we needed to move on before we potentially hurt each other and ruined our friendship.

Even in ending our relationship, we were in sync. (And also 'N Sync since we had a shared obsession for 90s pop music, but that's another story).

Damian's still my best friend now and he's godfather to my two children. I was also a witness at his wedding and we still holiday together to this day.

We made the right decision and thank goodness we did because few relationships get to where ours has.

After breaking up with Damian, I bought my first home

by myself. It was a one bed, teeny, tiny apartment in Leeds city centre and oh, how I loved that flat.

Turning the key every day when I came home made my heart sing. It was my sanctuary, my bubble where I could continue to work on finding out who I was supposed to be.

This time, there was no broken heart to mend and Damian even helped me move in and he came around for dinner regularly.

It felt so 'grown up' and it was.

My second time as a singleton - age twenty-five.

It's 2003 and I am living the single girl dream.

I dictate what I do all day and every day. I'm working in recruitment in a job I love and with colleagues I adore.

Being a recruiter suits me splendidly and I'm bloody good at it. I'm the highest biller my office has had in a while, my clients rate me and I'm earning a small fortune.

Designer handbags and European mini breaks are now monthly occurrences and I'm loving life.

Except on Sundays, when being single is a bit shit. Long drives out to countryside pubs and snuggles on the sofa are scarce. But one day of 'meh' when the rest of the week rocks is more than doable.

Being single at age twenty-five was different though because I was one of a few singletons in my circle of friends.

Thankfully for me, Niamh had been dumped again (sorry Niamh!). Our relationships strangely always started and ended at around the same time. Her heart wasn't broken either and despite her living in Manchester, we met up regularly for drunken nights out and lazy wine-fuelled lunches.

I had two other single buddies, Kara and Sasha, who both lived in Leeds.

Every Friday and Saturday night, we'd hit the town, drink ourselves silly and dance on bar tops until 5am.

Despite the horrendous hangovers and hit to my bank balance, there were no horror stories to tell of this period of my life. Well, none I can recall.

I was earning a lot in my demanding job and loved being a sole homeowner. That flat was my little sanctuary.

From waking up every morning in a big bed to myself to turning the key after a long day at work, it was all mine. I was living my life to the full.

In the two years I was single again, and I know it's a cliché, but I discovered myself.

I found strengths I didn't know I had, and the world was my oyster.

But cracks appeared that I hadn't yet seen.

Heading to burnout - age twenty-six.

In my waking hours I was doing one of two things; working or drinking.

I mean, there were trips to see the family and other more normal activities scattered in between but work and partying occupied my days and nights.

When I moved into my flat, I had a rule I stuck to rigidly: I would never drink alcohol alone. I think even then I knew if I started to, I'd be drinking alone every night and it wouldn't be healthy.

So, I only drank when I went out on Friday and Saturday nights.

But, over time, in my quest to fill my social calendar, and possibly to find a man, my weekends stretched out to include Thursday nights and Sunday afternoons too.

From after work on Thursday until I went to bed on a Sunday, I was drinking heavily.

With my elevated income, the alcopops had turned into champagne. And let's not forget the 'buy two large glasses of wine and get the rest of the bottle free' offer that was trending in UK bars at the time. I think they still do that.

Don't mind if I do. I LOVE to save money.

Work was busy and successful but stressful and my insomnia was at an all-time high.

On Sunday nights, knowing I had to get up early for work, I couldn't sleep. It wasn't because I didn't love my job; it was the pressure of only having six hours to cram in some sleep.

Then five hours, four, three, two, one, none.

I would clock watch all night with scattered minutes of light sleeping here and there and by Monday morning, I'd feel like a zombie.

Throughout the week, the insomnia would continue but out of pure exhaustion, I would find it easier and easier to get to sleep as the week went on.

Come Thursday or Friday, I felt the tiniest bit more human but then the nights out started again, and this cycle of heavy drinking and little sleep continued for months.

My job was highly competitive, and I was determined to be the best. I wasn't weighed down with partners and kids like my peers were and I could pour every second into the job.

So, when work emails came in at 10pm, I wouldn't leave responding to them until the next day, I'd deal with them immediately.

Checking my work Blackberry became an obsession and made me frantic.

High stress, no sleep, relentless drinking. It took its toll.

Sitting in the boardroom with my boss, I said, "I can't do this anymore" and cried. My head was on the desk at the time. It was dramatic.

I was knocking at the door of burn out and had to save myself.

A girl at work had returned from a six-month trip around the world and talked frequently about her travels, the places she visited and what it was like to work abroad.

She spoke with so much fire and passion and I wanted in.

Travelling the world had never appealing to me though. By that I mean the whole back-packing thing. My idea of travel was five-star luxury hotels, and that's what I had hoped for more of in my future.

Working abroad though, that called to me. I love work; I love to see new places and I love to teach.

China was a country I had always longed to visit, and I investigated the possibility of taking some time off to work in China, teaching English at a Chinese school or orphanage.

The more I researched the trip, the more places I wanted to see, and the trip quickly turned into a plan to see more of South East Asia. It was cheaper to travel 'around the world' than go to Asia and back so I tagged

Australia on to my plans too.

The thought of taking such a big leap terrified me but you know who else was about to take six months off to travel the world? Damian was.

Damian and his new girlfriend, who I'd met a couple of times and seemed lovely. If you were hoping for a rekindling of romance, think again!

My friend, Marie, was about to start on her travels too.

The timing was eerily perfect, and it seemed to be the best mix of solo travel, working abroad and having best friends from home to meet up with along the way.

Leaving the UK and finding a husband - age twenty-seven.

I didn't quit my job but took a six-month sabbatical although in my mind I hoped I wouldn't return.

Hong Kong was one place I booked to travel to and had been a place I had been considering looking for work in. The global business I worked for had offices in most countries so it would be an easy move to be transferred.

On October 14th, 2017, I set off to my first stop, China. My intentions for the trip were simple: see the world, work abroad and kiss a man in each country I visited. What can I say, I'm driven by goals and I know what I want!

But I didn't want the trip to only be about sight-seeing and fun times. I wanted to find a purpose too and I had an open mind to whether I would even return to the UK and to my job. I knew somehow this trip would lead to *something new*.

I had researched online and found an orphanage in Xi'an, China who were looking for volunteers to work for them and help look after disabled babies. I hadn't finished the first paragraph when I knew it was the project for me. Something instinctively told me I could make a difference by doing this work—for those children and for me too.

I started in China and then planned to travel to Thailand, Malaysia, Singapore, Australia and New Zealand.

On my second day in Beijing, China I'd met up with a group of volunteers who would join me in Xi'an on different volunteer projects. It just happened we would be all arriving in Beijing first.

I had started a travel blog to journal my trip for people back home and I wrote about meeting up with the group and how excited I was about it.

We caught up with everyone at Tiananmen Square as it was central. We'd then go for dinner. One of the group members, Tim, had said he was bringing a friend he'd met on the Great Wall of China that day. As you do.

I wrote in my blog, wondering if Tim's friend would be, well, 'hot'. That's probably what I said at the time - it was a long time ago. Turns out, he wasn't.

He wasn't my type at all. He was quiet, wore a hoodie with skulls on it and had his head down most of the time. How annoying.

He was Australian, but he didn't watch Neighbours *or* Home and Away.

He was in Beijing on holiday from the Philippines where he was working on a contract as an animator with Disney. I didn't like Disney.

I wrote in my blog what a letdown he was but never mind, plenty more fish in all the seas I was about to see.

The next day a few of us met up again for a day trip to the Hutongs and then at night to see a Chinese acrobatics show which was amazing. He came along again. I'm sure he had the same clothes on. Such an effort.

That night we went for dinner and most of the group went home after that. I stayed out with Katie, one girl in the group, and the Aussie.

We went to a dodgy club in the city and it was a bit of a weird night. We made the most of it, had a few drinks and hopped in a taxi home in the early hours.

As the taxi pulled up to my hotel, the Aussie asked if he'd be getting out too and coming in with me. Hold up, what?

However, a few cocktails in, I'd decided he might be worth a 'pash' so that's what happened in the taxi. For the record, I'm yet to hear an actual Aussie call a kiss a 'pash' but play along with me.

Our eyes met, our lips locked, and our teeth bashed into each other. Twice. It wasn't awful, but it certainly wasn't earth moving. The taxi driver cringed for us. Because yes, he'd turned around in his seat for the show. I excused myself and went inside.

Oh well, despite the crap kiss, I could check off kissing a man in China. He was Australian but details.

A week later I was in Xi'an and loving working at the orphanage, but something wasn't right. My heart hurt. It just *hurt* and I couldn't understand why. I met up with Marie and talked to her about it, confessing whilst I didn't know why, I missed this man.

I didn't find him as interesting, captivating or anything I thought I would when I met "The One" but I really, really missed him. Despite the amazing opportunity I was so enjoying.

When my project was ending, I was set to visit Hong Kong next and then Thailand. I'd started Facebook messaging the Aussie at this point and he'd invited me to the Philippines in the few days I had spare between Hong Kong and Thailand.

Now on Facebook, he was so much more fun. In fact, what a flirtatious, hilarious keyboard warrior he was!

I was weighing up whether to go to the Philippines, Vietnam or Cambodia. I'd heard awesome things about the latter two, but one needed a visa and the other had no flights. So, I booked tickets to Manila and slowly started to look forward to going. More than anything, I wanted to stop my heart from hurting and I wondered if seeing the Aussie would get it out of my system.

Had I somehow romanticised he was something he wasn't?

I wanted to know if this man meant anything at all to me or if I could forget about him and enjoy the rest of my trip. So off I went to Hong Kong until the day I boarded the plane to Manila.

He didn't meet me at the airport. I instead was conned into a magical mystery tour of the city by a cheeky taxi driver. I finally reached my hotel in Makati. The Aussie had invited me to stay at his place but there was no way that was happening. So, I settled on a hotel in the business district, thinking I'd be staying with other corporate types.

Upon checking in, they gave me my room swipe key

and a voucher for a free drink at the bar. *Interesting*... but I do love a free drink.

I threw my backpack in the room and headed to the bar for the freebie, waiting for the Aussie to text me back and tell me where to meet him for drinks that night. I went back to my room and annoyingly, my key card had stopped working. A hotel worker in the hallway came over to let me in. What a nice friendly man he was. Until he told me he could get into my room at any time. Um, argh.

I called the Aussie who insisted on coming to collect me immediately so we could find somewhere else for me to stay. Such chivalry! Out we checked and off we went to a local bar to chat.

A few drinks in I decided he presented much less of a risk than the psycho hotel worker so, I agreed to sleep on his sofa.

I was never going to sleep on his sofa.

What I mean is, I would make *him* sleep on his sofa and I'd sleep in the bed.

How exciting though, I then had a kiss in the Philippines. Same man but again, details.

The next day we went to the internet cafe in his building so I could upload some pics to my Facebook page. We were already 'Facebook friends' but I told him I would make him my Facebook 'boyfriend' for a laugh to see if my friends at home commented on it. He told me to go for it, so I did. Oh, how we laughed! Actually, we forgot about it and went for lunch.

My next stop would be Bangkok where I'd also be meeting Damian and May (his girlfriend) who were there at the same time. It would have been my 28th birthday by then so I had a big night out in mind for when we reunited.

After a couple of days, the Aussie asked me to stay longer and spend my birthday with him instead and after a lot of indecisiveness; I did. I wanted to spend more time with him. He was so much more fun than I had imagined and let's not forget; we were Facebook official.

When I was with him, my heart no longer hurt.

Side note: at this point I'd told my parents I had an *actual* boyfriend and while it disappointed them that 1) he didn't live in England and 2) he had a tattoo; they were delighted I was no longer "on the shelf". Bit rude.

So, I celebrated my birthday in Manila with the Aussie, my ex and his girlfriend who had joined us there instead. As you do.

After another few days I finally boarded the plane to Bangkok and sobbed like a baby from the moment I kissed the Aussie goodbye. It was at this point I realised that 99% of my iPod was made up of sad, broken heart songs. It didn't help.

This time, my heart didn't just hurt, it almost broke. I had no idea when or if I'd see him again and despite looking forward to all the travel plans I had ahead, I just Felt. So. Sad.

There I was in Thailand with my ex, his girlfriend and his Mum. She'd come over for a holiday for a couple of weeks. We're all very close, ok? I invited the Aussie over for a weekend and he said yes.

He'd finished his contract and was heading back to Australia for good but came to see me first. We had an awesome weekend together in Bangkok where again, I ticked off a 'let's kiss a man in each country' check box. I've always hit my targets.

Sadness followed again as he headed home, but I had Christmas and New Year on Koh Phangan to look forward to. In fact, that Christmas was still my favourite one ever. Before kids, of course.

I'd spent six weeks in Thailand getting qualified in Thai massage (a skill I've never since used), playing in the sea, drinking cocktails on the beach and going to Full Moon parties.

I was missing the Aussie though and my phone bill of £450 in one month proved that. So, when he asked if I wanted to change my plans and head to Australia a few weeks earlier, I followed my heart and went.

I never went to Malaysia or Singapore, something I regret, but I always believe in following your heart and gut instinct.

We had a brilliant time in Sydney bringing in the New Year together and with some of his friends and family. In fact, a few days later I headed with him to his hometown and met his *entire* family.

The Aussie and I were a couple, on Facebook and in real life. He asked me to move to Australia and to give our relationship a real go and I didn't hesitate in saying yes. I just *knew* it was the right thing to do and a risk worth taking. In fact, it didn't feel like a risk at all.

We headed back to the UK to pack up my things, rent out my apartment and emigrate to Australia.

My sabbatical was for six months but three months in, I'd completed a life-changing volunteer project, met some amazing people, seen some of the world, met "The One" and immigrated to Australia.

I hadn't missed out on everything. Let's not forget I'd achieved my ultimate goal of kissing a man in every country I visited, and I could now add Australia and the UK to that list.

I suppose I could add Malaysia and Singapore too if you count the airports for our connecting flights.

I sometimes think of those moments when I might not have followed my heart. If we hadn't had the bad first kiss in Beijing. If I hadn't gone to the Philippines. Or if we hadn't decided so quickly to put our relationship out there for the world to see (on Facebook). Well, it could have been very different.

He still wears that skull hoodie. I dislike it.

But since then, we've married twice (in Australia and the UK) and had two beautiful babies.

I'm not a believer in there being only one person in the world who is right for you. I believe there are many 'ones'.

My first two relationships were not perfect, but they were close in many ways too.

My present relationship isn't always perfect but over a decade on, we still madly and passionately love each other and have so much in common.

We've always been a social couple but we're also happy having a night in together, even before the kids.

Drinking alcohol has always been a big part of our lives; whether it's a romantic dinner and a bottle of wine or a holiday in the Hunter Valley vineyards.

We've thrown many parties over the years, had some amazing weekends away with friends and have a shared passion for karaoke. All fuelled by copious amounts of alcohol, of course.

Our drinking was pretty well-matched although I was the driving force behind opening most bottles.

My own heavy drinking continued throughout my late twenties and early thirties.

Alcohol fuelled nights that, in the main, did not induce vomiting or embarrassing incidents. Just almighty hangovers, shameful apologies and a deep-rooted paranoia of 'what the hell did I do last night?'

That got to me more than the physical symptoms. The worry and guilt I might have shown myself up, upset someone or done something I might regret.

It's played on my mind many times over the years. The morning after the day before, I could almost always pinpoint the time in the evening where I should have stopped drinking but didn't.

The tipping point. The time I needed to rein myself in, or have someone else say "right, that's it, no more wine for you!" and pass me the water or take me home.

I wouldn't have listened or left though.

Trying for a baby - aged thirty-four.

It's 2012, we're newly married and having a baby is at the top of our "what we'll conquer next" list.

However, getting pregnant wasn't as easy as we expected. It took a few months or more of hard core trying. You know, everything from ovulation tests with smiley faces, to timing of The Sex to pillows under hips and legs in the air.

I mean, if I'd known I wasn't going to become instantly pregnant, I might not have spent so much time in my early twenties lying awake thinking I might be up the duff. Don't tell my daughter I said that. Or my son.

The sex wasn't the problem. I mean, there was plenty

of it at all times of the day and night because you can't be too accurate when planning ovulation apparently and we wanted to cover all ovulation bases. However, my stress levels rose and with every trip to the loo that resulted in a monthly "Hey Bitch, I'm BAAACK!" from Aunt Flo. I grew more and more concerned something wasn't right and perhaps motherhood wasn't for me. It ripped me apart and despite getting excited about our honeymoon approaching, it was always on my mind.

We'd decided to have our honeymoon six months after the wedding so we had something else to look forward to. Well, it's all over in a flash otherwise, isn't it?

In those six months, the wedding diet went slightly out of the window and my consumption of cheap wine rose.

My two best friends, Damian and May, moved over from the UK and lived with us whilst they were setting themselves up with jobs and their own apartment.

It was the best of times. It was the drunkest of times. It was fun!

But there was no baby, and it tugged at my heart.

When we finally set off for our 9-night Bali adventure, it was the holiday we desperately needed.

We decided on the plane journey over that for us, 'adventure' translated to sun loungers and cocktails. However, when we got to our beautiful private villa (which had its own private pool, peeps!) getting smashed on booze was the last thing on our minds.

We slept in, ate fresh food, drank very little and had early nights. It was bliss. Utter indulgence and the time to relax and chill with each other that we so desperately needed after the whirlwind of the wedding.

During the trip, my period was late and, being a romantic at heart, I bought a pregnancy test from the pharmacy. I mean, imagine finding out I was pregnant whilst on honeymoon. How special would that be? Not special as it happens, not pregnant.

I was getting used to false tests by now so picked myself up quickly and we enjoyed the rest of our trip. Another period came and went, when we got back.

Getting home, back to reality, was a bump to say the least after such a beautiful and blissful break. But this was the start of the rest of our married lives and we were excited to be buying a house together soon. We were on the lookout for the perfect one, in fact.

A few weeks after we returned from our honeymoon, we hosted a Christmas in July party at home and invited a few close friends over to celebrate.

That morning I was excited to get the flat ready. It was a week before my period was due but, my body was telling me to do a pregnancy test. Hell, my nipples were practically opening the test packet.

POSITIVE.

The faintest of faint pink lines appeared on the test and I sat on the toilet in amazement. Just like they do on the telly.

"I don't see anything," my husband said.

I took approximately 1,254,567 more tests.

"I do! I see the line!" May screamed.

They had just moved out of our flat but had come around to set up for the party.

"Nah," said Damian.

But there were two pink lines. Two of them. I saw. May

saw. And after a while, the husband agreed too. Fucking hell.

It's a weird feeling, when you're desperately trying to get pregnant and then finally find out you are.

A what-the-hell-how-did-this-happen-have-I-made-a-mistake-oh-my-God-I'm-so-excited-I-might-burst kind of feeling.

And I suppose that would mean no wine for me tonight.

But I was three weeks pregnant—only THREE weeks. And we didn't want anyone to know, so I had to clutch the same glass of warm red wine all night in the hope no one would notice I wasn't drinking any of it. They didn't, thankfully.

A healthy first trimester followed and at twelve weeks, we announced to the world baby Jenkinson was en route.

I didn't drink alcohol through either of my pregnancies. For me, the risk to my child wasn't worth it and as I've pointed out before, I've always been 'all or nothing' when it came to drinking anyway.

My pregnancy was fairly trouble free, and for eight months and three weeks I drank no alcohol, ate healthily and even partook in prenatal Pilates.

Then, after thirty-six weeks and six days, my beautiful bouncing baby girl arrived, and we were a happy family of three!

My first drink after I became a mum - aged thirty-five.

I remember my first drink after having my first baby. We'd taken her to meet our friends, and they'd cracked open a bottle of wine to celebrate.

As a breastfeeding mother, who had survived on next to no sleep during that first two weeks of motherhood, I agreed to the tiniest splash of wine in my glass. I wanted to be social and celebrate but had no interest in drinking.

Even that sip, which was barely that, felt like it hit my brain immediately, making me feel woozy. And that was the last time I touched alcohol for a while.

The first few months of motherhood were the toughest of my life. I felt the pressure of being at home with a baby by myself, having no support or family nearby and barely any sleep.

I wouldn't call her a cat-napper as I think cats sleep longer than twenty minutes at a time, don't they? But that's what she did: twenty minutes at a time day and night.

When she fed, it was a ninety-minute lazy lunch. All I did was feed her and then pace with her upright for hours on end. She would not let me sit down, not even to perch on the back of the sofa.

We were exhausted, and we were at breaking point but then, one night at around ten-weeks-old, she slept.

It had been slowly creeping up, I think. She slept for a little longer each session and awoke fewer times throughout the night. That one magical night, she slept for eight hours in a row.

When we awoke, and it was daylight and not midnight, we leapt out of bed to her cot to make sure she was still breathing. She couldn't possibly have SLEPT. But she had, and that was the start of a much easier spell of sleep for the whole family.

Six months later, I started weaning my daughter, ready to return to work. At that point, she'd been sleeping through the night for some time too and we reintroduced alcohol into some of our evenings.

It built up over time and I even had the occasional girls' night out too. This meant catching up with friends, staying out late and being able to eat a full meal, uninterrupted, whilst it was still hot.

It also meant a lot of wine and a few cocktails for good measure.

My alcohol tolerance levels were low in the beginning but the more regularly I drank, well, the more I drank.

The 7pm "Mummy Wine Time" Habit.

Despite the sleepless start to motherhood, it got much easier as time went on.

In fact, both of my babies loved their sleep. Let me add this is no longer the case and they've decided sleeping is for chumps.

But even now, by 7pm every night they're tucked up in bed and fast asleep. At least until midnight and sometimes straight through until 7am as they did for years before now.

For us, this meant victory and every good 'win' deserves to be celebrated, right?

We'd cracked Parenting. None of our friends' kids slept as well as ours. None of them followed the bedtime routines as easily as our kids did.

As much as we sometimes missed being able to go out at night with friends, we enjoyed each other's company and loved nothing more than a night in front of the telly together, uninterrupted. That was more than enough for us.

Even then, most Friday and Saturday nights, you'd find the two of us on the sofa in front of Netflix with a takeout in one hand and a large glass of wine in the other.

Sometimes, my husband didn't drink. He didn't always seem to *need* the wine like I did.

And whilst I had a rule throughout my life I'd never drink alone, sometimes I'd crack open the wine when he wasn't drinking. He was in the same room, that was still social, right?

As the weeks and months went on, that 7pm 'fix' became a more regular occurrence.

Sunday night wine time crept in and, because I worked for myself at home, I didn't need to get to an office. I mean, getting up with the kids was sometimes a struggle but if I didn't wash my hair that day, no one would notice at school drop-off time.

Working for myself gave me so much flexibility when planning my days—and nights.

Thursdays joined the mix and soon we were both drinking one to two bottles per night between us, four nights a week.

But then, on a Monday, we might end the day with a glass or three too. Well, Mondays are hard, aren't they? No one who works likes Mondays, do they?

You need to wind down on a Monday and isn't wine awesome for that feeling of instant relaxation?

Then there are Wednesdays. Well, they're hump days, aren't they? And you know what hump days are? They're 'happy'. Cheers, Happy Hump Day!

Drinking more regularly didn't happen overnight and slowly increased over a few years.

We relocated temporarily to the UK, and I had my second baby there.

But over time, and especially in the past couple of years, drinking alcohol most nights a week became something we just *did*.

Some weeks, three nights. Some weeks, every night.

Let's not forget, I'd cultivated the habit of drinking a lot from a young age. I'd fought past tolerance levels, outdrank my opponents and battled the anxiety-driven monsters. All alcoholic achievements unlocked. I was up-levelling to dependency.

Of course, I was fighting monsters with monsters. I just didn't realise it at the time.

My consumption of alcohol hasn't all led to embarrassing outcomes and I won't bore you with the details of all the grim, humiliating times I've had ten too many.

But in the past twenty-plus years since I started drinking, I'd been able to hold my own on many occasions. To have a few glasses of wine, or even a few bottles across a weekend bender, and act appropriately.

No vomit, no embarrassing outbursts, many nights of dancing on tables and karaoke sessions that have been perfectly harmless and drama-free.

I suppose I'm lucky humiliation, shame and the occasional day of retching has been my greatest punishment for the amount of alcohol I've drunk over the years.

My liver has survived the abuse I've thrown upon it.

I've drunk at work functions, weddings, charity events and family parties and my alcohol consumption hasn't appeared to have had any negative impact whatsoever.

I've worked in corporate jobs for most of my life. As a non-tea and coffee drinker, I would joke from day one of my new job it was only 'water and wine' for me. Such a bad Brit, quite antisocial of me.

Having a handy excuse from making the entire team a cup of tea numerous times a day was a definite pro. But I was always first to offer a round at the bar on an office night out.

For most of my life, I've been the one who has spent hours comforting a drunk, over-emotional friend, holding back another's hair or ensuring another gets home safely or puts the drink down.

I'm the reliable friend. The one everyone else can count on for common sense, comfort and security.

I'm the life of the party, the agony aunt, the truth teller and the life coach. The one who has their shit together.

I can also always be relied on as a drinking buddy, night out organiser, karaoke partner, cocktail-swigger and the one who always ensured we would get home safely.

Starting a family reduced the amount of times these events happened significantly, of course, but when I was out, I was *out.*

My cancer diagnosis - aged thirty-six.

It's 2015 and I've been happily married for three years. I'd just moved back to Australia with my husband, two-year-old daughter and five-month-old son.

I'd had my second baby in the UK, again after some months of trying and thinking it would never happen until the happy day it did.

We'd been living in the UK for eighteen months on a working holiday, spending time with family and enjoying the last time we would be back there for a while.

After deciding on a date to come back to Australia, we found an apartment in Newcastle, NSW. I started a great job and we were excited about my parents moving over from the UK, too.

Our family was complete, and we were planning to buy our forever home. You know, the house we would raise our babies in and create beautiful memories as our happy family of four. It was going to be a-mazing.

We could unpack our things for the last time ever and get our finances in order to provide for the kids and plan our next holiday.

A week or so into the new job, I was showering before work and felt a lump in my left breast. *What the hell was that?*

Grapelike in size, it was hard and painless.

As I was weaning my baby son from breastfeeding, I assumed the lump was probably a blocked milk duct and frantically tried to massage it out.

It didn't break up or loosen, and in fact, my rubbing it made it quite sore.

I'm a proactive and extremely impatient person and rang to make an appointment with a new GP that morning. My lovely new boss let me have time off to go when I explained the situation.

How embarrassing though. The second week into the

job and already I was taking time off. Not the positive and professional start I intended to make.

My new GP, another Brit in Aus., told me I'd done the right thing by getting it checked but he was also inclined to think it was a blocked duct.

That said, he thought it important to be sure and referred me for an ultrasound and, if needed, a mammogram.

The mammogram was needed apparently, and after both scans, I sat in the cold waiting room, wrapped in a too-small gown. Then the nurse came in to tell me they had arranged for me to have a biopsy in a few days.

"Why, what did you see?" I asked. Poker-faced, she gave nothing away. Nothing.

I chose not to panic. I'm a person who stresses about shit things when they *actually* happen, not just because they *might*. That was me then, anyway.

The biopsy wasn't too painful but took some time and a doctor came in part way through to examine the screen. Again, they gave me nothing. Although I remember their faces were quite un-smiley.

Days went by and I called my doctor's office constantly but was told the results hadn't come back yet. Days.

I decided I would have been contacted immediately if it was a problem. They'd never let me carry on as normal if I had actual cancer, right?

I'd almost given up even calling them, but my boss told me to try one more time.

Sat in a meeting room at work, I picked up the phone and called the surgery. As I was put through to the nurse, I took a deep breath and asked if my results were back.

"The Doctor would like you to come in to talk about the results," she said.

Oh, holy fuck. *Those* words. Those ones. Like off the TV.

"It's cancer, isn't it?" The words escaped my mouth.

"Can you come in now?" she said.

"Yes," I whispered.

As tears streamed down my face, I ended the call and immediately phoned my husband. The kids were at their new day care centre and he was at home, a few minutes away, applying for jobs.

"You have to come here right now, and we have to go to the doctors right now and I have cancer and so you have to come here right now, ok?" I told him in one breath.

"What, what?" he said.

But he came, and we walked the ten minutes to the GP's office. Silent, holding hands tightly. Internally crying.

"You have Triple Negative Breast Cancer," the GP said.

Not the original GP. This one was a kindly Australian woman who looked at me with such sympathy. My GP was away.

"What the fuck is that?" I said, minus the F word because she looked nice and I try my best not to swear at nice strangers. Especially doctors, etc.

Apparently, Triple Negative Breast Cancer is a rare and aggressive 'treat' of a cancer. It has no failsafe cure and 'they' don't seem to know what causes it.

Oh good, I've always wanted to be a bit quirky. Brilliant.

Would I have to have a mastectomy? Yes. *Chemo?* Yes. And radiation. Oh.

My 'forever home', complete family, happy life was vanishing before my eyes.

All I could imagine was the life I might now never have.

My kids starting school.

Dancing at their weddings.

Holding my first grandchild.

How did I get cancer? Did I cause this? What did I do wrong?

I met the man who would be my surgeon that week and, after assessing my results, he said I wouldn't need a mastectomy after all. I would have a lumpectomy to remove the lump, then chemo and radiation.

My 37th birthday was the very next day.

Would I ever get to be an old person? I might not even make it to forty.

But a feeling of optimism flooded me and after sharing what was happening with my family, friends and blog readers, I felt uplifted and full of hope.

Shit scared, but hopeful.

As the weeks and months passed, I underwent surgery to remove the lump and then treatment. And I'll take a moment to acknowledge gratitude the lump had found a home in my left breast, the significantly larger of the two.

So, whilst my boobs are now a little wonky, they are generally more even than they were before. #winning

A brave new world.

I'm a confident woman but many things scare me. You know, flying, drowning, spiders, heights, bananas.

Yes, bananas. *shudder*

Death though, is the biggest thing that scares me and I'm sure I'm not alone in being most scared of my own death or that of a family member dying.

But facing a cancer diagnosis that made me feel like I might die on the spot, suddenly, I felt brave. I mean, it was happening. I was going to die, and a lot sooner than I'd planned.

But what else was there to fear? I tried to block the repercussions of my dying from my mind. The impact on my family, my babies.

I suppose I became more confident about what I wanted and didn't want in my life anymore though.

No more tolerating fools or foolish decisions. In the limited time I had left, I was no longer prepared to waste it on the things and people that didn't count. It was strangely liberating and a feeling I wished I'd had and embraced years before.

Family and friends rallied around me and I had never felt more loved, supported and wanted.

I didn't always feel all-powerful though and over time, this waned.

Chemotherapy, as it happens, was worse than I could have ever imagined. During the six months I endured it, I lost my hair, some friends and almost my mind.

Turns out some friends are only there for the fair-weather days and cancer places itself, and therefore you, into the 'too hard basket'.

Yes, some friends deserted me, and some showed their less-than-friendly side. I suppose I still feel some resentment towards them but again; it was quite liberating knowing I could cut people out of my life if they no longer added anything positive to it.

I have never felt as physically ill in my life as during this time and hope never to again. I wouldn't wish chemo on my worst enemy and despite being hopeful it was for the greater good, and having faith in its ability to cure me, I resented it.

When my treatment ended though, it surprised me how quickly I began returning to my old self. In some ways, but certainly not all.

My hair started to slowly grow, and my grey pallor regained a little more glow.

But inside, I was utterly broken. I was a shattered, damaged version of the woman I once was.

I was also heavier. 10kgs to be exact. I looked in the mirror and didn't see myself looking back. To be honest, I didn't feel particularly female and certainly not attractive.

Throughout chemo, when I lost my hair, I would stare deeply into my own eyes in the mirror. I told myself whatever happened around them, those eyes were still mine. I was still there, inside.

Before chemo, I'd assumed that weight would fall off me. "This is going to be the best enforced diet ever!" I joked to my friends with a fake smile plastered on my face.

But no, during chemo the steroids stopping me from throwing up made me balloon and crave carbs. And all sorts of craziness happened to my hormones.

But overall, I felt elated the worst was over, and I could try to get back to normal living. My new, old life.

Part of getting back to normal was allowing some of my old habits to creep back in.

The hubs and I had become accustomed to putting the

kids to bed, sitting in front of Netflix and cracking open a bottle of wine.

Generally, we shared that one bottle. And generally, it was on a Friday and Saturday night.

For years, we both had to get up early for work and then for early rising kids. We soon learned hangovers don't mix well with that.

But during most of my treatment, we were both working reduced hours.

My parents had come over from the UK and moved in with us to help look after my kids when I was at appointments or too sick to do much. And, of course, to look after me, their daughter.

When I could, I worked from home on my blog which had changed from a hobby blog to a place where I could collaborate with brands to earn an income.

I also shared my whole journey with cancer and treatment, and my life as a busy mum. You can read my blog at <u>lovefrommim.com</u>.

Working from home gave me flexibility and a much-needed income to help pay off the medical bills we had racked up and the debts from neither of us being in work.

The flexibility meant I could spend more time with my kids and having my parents help me gave me so much freedom.

It felt like a holiday from *real* life and after what I'd been through; I deserved a holiday.

And what do many people do when they're on holiday? They indulge. I did.

I started to drink again during the end of my treatment when the effects of the chemo drugs had worn off. And you know what I discovered, I no longer had hangovers.

Nothing.

I couldn't decide if it was a side effect of chemo (I have an endless list of other side effects). Or because I felt so ill during chemo, I might never feel anything like that bad ever again.

But, anyway, no hangovers? What? Well, that was something worth celebrating. With wine.

The frequency and quantity I drank went up and down over the next year or so as I slowly adjusted to being cancer-free and out of treatment.

A year later, my business had three different income streams, and I mainly earned money from advertisers who would sponsor articles on my blog.

I also freelanced as a writer and social media manager for other businesses and had a small online shop making and selling planner stickers.

The common denominator was 'time' and making the best use of my time and helping others to make time for themselves.

So, whether it was the mums who read my blog articles, the clients I worked for or the customers who used my planners and stickers to be more organised, I was helping others to find more time for the things that meant the most to them.

I realised there was a need for me, and my skill set, and it surprised me how many requests I had for help. I mean, I knew in my heart my business would be successful, but it shocked me when it started to happen.

My income increased and, over time, my reputation grew, and more opportunities came in.

My one year 'all-clear' appointment rolled in, then two years, three and more.

But whilst celebrating occurred publicly, I had not mended the broken pieces inside.

I started to see a psychologist and talked with them for hours, pouring my heart out about the deep fear I had about the cancer coming back and me not being here for my children.

I desperately wanted to live a full life without fear, but I couldn't seem to throw myself headfirst into it.

I was grateful but stunted. Held back. So very frightened. And then, anxious.

My first experience with Anxiety - aged thirty-seven.

Throughout my life, I've encountered people with anxiety, but I never truly understood what it was.

Beyond Blue defines anxiety as "more than just feeling stressed or worried. Whilst stress and anxious feelings are a common response to a situation where we feel under pressure, they usually pass once the stressful situation has passed, or 'stressor' is removed.

Anxiety is when these anxious feelings don't go away, when they're ongoing and happen without any reason or cause. It's a serious condition that makes it hard to cope with daily life. Everyone feels anxious from time to time, but for someone experiencing anxiety, these feelings aren't easily controlled."

Before I knew what anxiety really was, I identified it as a friend who suffered from depression and took medication every day.

Or a friend who had panic attacks and sometimes couldn't leave the house.

Or those who drank or took drugs to excess to face the day.

Nervous people, those with anger issues, OCD. You know, *they* had anxiety.

Now, I knew better.

Although I was often an awkward teen or an insecure twenty-something woman, I don't think I was ever particularly anxious.

As I got older, my confidence grew and I determined much more easily who I was, what I wanted and the woman I wanted to be.

Cancer messed all of that up. Depression. Emptiness. Living in fear.

Since the day they diagnosed me, my life changed forever. Suddenly my whole world was tipped upside down. Everything I had, my whole life and the life of my family, was under threat. Fear set in quickly.

I was determined to beat cancer. To complete my treatment. It wasn't easy. In fact, chemotherapy was, without a doubt, the worst period of my entire life. I felt alone, confused and so very unwell.

It wasn't all bad. I now had this newfound confidence in saying 'No' to things that no longer served me.

I no longer wasted time on rubbish friends who sapped my energy and gave nothing back.

I turned down work that wasn't in line with my long-term goals.

I no longer took any crap from anyone. I felt powerful. Cancer had strengthened me, and made me more resilient, unstoppable.

But also, so very fearful. And no one had the answers to appease my fears, to address them or crush them.

"Live every day like it's your last!" I'm frequently told. "Stay positive and it will all be ok!"

Shut up!

I mean, they mean so well, but I *am* positive. But I was positive before I got cancer and I still *got* cancer.

Every good appointment I had and every positive scan and test result that came back was amazing. It was like being given my life back to me as a great gift. So, while I dreaded, and still dread, some of my medical appointments, I knew how wonderfully positive I would feel when the results came back as good.

Another chance. A bit more time.

But what about the depression, the emptiness and living in fear? Would that be forever? Would I live with fear forever?

I was petrified and had visions of being told the cancer has come back.

I thought about cancer every single day.

There are times when I forgot but then would hear bad news from others. A new diagnosis, or a cancer has returned, or someone has passed away.

In 2016, Facebook was a bloody nightmare for me to be on. Everyone seemed to joke about the spate of celebrity deaths. How tragic it was that so many 'greats' were passing away in the same year. Wasn't 2016 a horrible year?

Did you notice many of those celebrities unfortunately died of cancer? It broke my heart for them and their families. It broke my heart too to see the way the press, and my friends, debated it. Insensitively at times.

Would I be joining the doomed 2016 list?

And it compounded my fear. Because when you have cancer, it's everywhere. Even on Facebook.

Every time I walk into my doctor's office, I remember sitting while I received my diagnosis and what went through my head.

Songs that come on the radio take me back to the dark days. I'll likely always associate some of my favourite songs with those times.

I couldn't pick up and move on with my life in the way I wanted to. I knew the fear was rational, of course.

Sleeping tablets helped me quiet some of the night demons for a short time but I hated the groggy feeling the next day, so I stopped taking them.

But one loyal and long-standing friend had the answers I was looking for. This friend had been with me through all the ups, downs, failures and celebrations in my life from a young age and was still here now. They were patiently waiting for me to call and invite them over for a chat.

Alcohol.

My first award nomination - aged thirty-nine.

In mid-2018 I receive an email telling me I've been nominated for an award and my first reaction is that it's a hoax.

I've turned into a bit of a cynic in recent years, you see.

As it turns out, it's a 100% legit award for Australian

Mums in Business and I am absolutely and utterly bloody delighted!

In the past couple of years, I've poured my heart and soul into building up a successful business, delighting clients and earning an income for my family.

This feels like validation—validation I know I don't need but it's delightful anyway. Recognition for the hard work, long hours and anxious moments of 'Am I doing the right thing here?'

The awards, the AusMumpreneur Awards, are renowned and recognised awards across Australia and I hold some previous winners in the highest regard.

When they named me as a finalist for the NSW Business Excellence award, I was over the moon. I mean, I already knew I wouldn't win, but the opportunity to network and practice pitching and learn from the conference speakers was too good an opportunity to miss.

I pinched myself at having this opportunity land in my lap to attend the conference and pitch, in person, to a panel of judges.

So off I went to Melbourne, fancy-ass dress in hand, ready to network up a storm.

Hundreds of Australian Mums in Business attended the conference, but something compelled me to sit at the front of the room with three others. Mainly because I'd left my glasses at home but also, they looked like a friendly bunch.

Peace Mitchell and Katy Garner, the AusMum founders, were also sat at the front table and it gave me a chance to say hello in person before the whirlwind of the next few days began.

When the time came for my panel interview, I was

psyched.

I love interviews. LOVE THEM. I'm confident, articulate and have over a decade of professional interview training and experience to back me up.

I've never stuffed an interview up and, most of the time, I get the job. Even if I don't want it.

I'm great at interviews.

This interview, not so great. Their first question asked me what I did. Easy enough to respond to.

The second was along the lines of, "Why did you start your business?".

I began, as I had a million and one times before with, "Well, in late 2015 I was diagnosed with a rare and aggressive type of breast cancer."

I stopped. And then, I cried.

I burst into tears, held my hand over my mouth and died a thousand deaths.

How? Why? I'd told this story so many times and I was so proud of my achievements. I had so much to say and I was so excited to be there. I had rehearsed this, and I knew all the words and it was All. Too. Much.

And didn't those beautiful women on the panel look at me so kindly, offer reassuring words and tissues and were so utterly lovely, the tears kept coming.

I pulled myself together as much as I could and bumbled through the rest of the interview, getting in most of what I wanted to say but not with the same confidence I had planned.

I spoke of the clients I'd worked with, why they came back to me, how I'd grown my reputation, my plans for the future, how much I was earning. I mean, I talked a lot. But with intermittent tears.

I usually leave interviews feeling like superwoman but at that time, I left feeling deflated and let down. By myself, it was certainly no one else's fault.

I wanted a do-over, but it would be another twelve months before I had the chance to be interviewed, *if* I ever made the finals again.

Imposter syndrome shat all over me and gave me the stark realisation I was out of place. I had no business being here with these kick-ass, high-flying, going-places women who had their stuff together.

I headed back to my table and my three new friends had their own tales of how they could have done things differently.

But we held up our chins and enjoyed the rest of the conference before heading back to our hotel to primp and preen before the awards ceremony.

Despite the slight horror of the interview, I felt amazing. I'd been dieting for a few months prior, had lost weight, curled my hair just right and was wearing a dress I felt like a princess in.

A few hours later, when they announced my category's finalists and they featured my name too, I squee'd in excitement and squeezed the hand of a fellow nominee who was sat at my table.

When they called my name as the winner, my heart skipped a beat.

No flipping way. *What?* It felt like a joke. They'd made a mistake. Had they forgotten I was the blubbering mess candidate? Had they confused me with one of the all-together champs who deserved this more?

Well, apparently not because my table buddies snapped me out of my haze and told me to get my arse up and on to the stage to accept my award.

Now, I'm a bit of a daydreamer and I'd already played this out in my head weeks before.

I'd float on stage, hug Peace and Katy, and graciously recount to the audience my tragic-to-terrific tale of business success.

Didn't go to plan.

It wasn't a float; it was more of a what-the-fuck-is-happening-rabbit-in-headlights-skulk on to the stage.

I hugged the girls; I remembered to thank the event sponsors, and I looked around at the crowd who waited with bated breath for my acceptance speech.

Which basically consisted of more tears and talk of cancer and boobs. I don't think I mentioned my business once, and I certainly forgot to thank my husband and family.

Big oops but also big yay because I'd bloody won.

I've tried and failed since to articulate well enough how much winning the award meant to me. It goes way beyond recognition for business success.

Winning the award didn't just validate my existence in Australia's busy and competitive world of mums in business, it seemed to validate my actual existence. Aside from being a mum.

It came at a time when I felt on the cusp of a new beginning, a new life and a new successful path.

But I was so totally terrified of cancer returning I felt paralysed and in denial the life I was working towards was an actual possibility.

Standing on that stage, it was like someone had lifted me out of the hole and placed me back onto the path I was so fiercely pushed off back in 2015.

The scenery was different, but my path was back, and it came with a shiny gold award.

The cherry on the top was my conference tablemates winning awards in their categories too.

Over the next year, I took my job more seriously. A bit of 'high-flyer Mim' was back and more success ensued.

However, the cracks were still there and starting to show up more. And my already frequent drinking became even more so.

HOW I GOT ADDICTED

Having been a big drinker for so many years, I hadn't noticed how much that amount had crept up and up.

Not just the quantity of alcohol in each sitting, but the frequency I was cracking open the bottles and turning to alcohol too.

In many of the appointments with my psychologist, I've mentioned how much I wanted to reduce the amount I was drinking and was honest about my consumption.

Before she could even suggest me giving up alcohol altogether, I got in first with a "I don't want to be teetotal, I just want to cut back."

We spoke a lot about my reasoning for this and I suppose I saw people who didn't drink as missing out. It wasn't so much I assumed they were boring or less fun than me. It's more I saw myself as *more* interesting and *more* fun when I drank, I suppose. So, I thought they were missing out on the potential to be better people because they were not drinking alcohol. How crazy is that? And judgemental.

So how much was I drinking? I've been loath to share the amount for two reasons.

First, you might be shocked and think badly of me. I mean, it's embarrassing.

The second reason for withholding the amount and frequency I was drinking is because I worry you won't see this is relative to *me* and *my* life.

What if you see the numbers and that makes you feel better about how much you are drinking? And if you also have a problem, what if you measure yourself up to me and don't acknowledge it?

Or you might be totally ok with drinking the same, or even more, than I was, and you might think I'm judging you.

What if you're in a similar position and me sharing my issue results in you feeling shame? Like I'm pointing the finger and saying, "Anyone who drinks this much, or more is a dirty, out-of-control lush who needs help and is addicted to alcohol." What if you think that? I would hate it to come across that way. It isn't my intention or belief.

The last thing I want to do is to put labels on anyone else. Only you know if you are in control or not of any aspect of your life. I'm not here to judge, name call or make you feel bad about yourself.

That said, if I didn't share the amount I was drinking, it wouldn't put some other things I talk about into perspective.

So, somewhat fearfully, I'll share it now. I was drinking 1-1.5 bottles of wine to myself almost every night.

Why was I drinking that much? Well, to get drunk. And by drunk, I mean to escape.

Because being drunk means I'm no longer afraid.

Good day at work? I opened the wine.

Bad day at work? Wine.

Scan result came back clear. Cheers to that!

Is that a new lump in my breast? I won't sleep tonight unless I have a drink.

What's that pain? Oh, it's your birthday! The new Outlander is out, let's watch it. It's Friday. It's Wednesday. It's 7pm and the kids are asleep.

And that last one has been the habit I have spent many hours forging over the last few years.

My kids have always been good sleepers. They fall to sleep easily and quickly and, if they get up in the night to come into bed with us, it's usually after midnight.

For many parents, this would be utter bliss. They can have a full evening to themselves, perhaps have an early night, and wake up early feeling refreshed and tackle whatever parenthood throws them that day.

That was me for a good while. Ask my friends. I SHOUTED about the fact my kids slept. Parenting? I had that shit sorted.

But instead of spending those evenings at the gym, tidying the house, having an early night or even writing the book I've longed to write since I was a teen, I drank.

One glass on the odd night turned into two glasses, three, more nights, all nights.

Over the years, I cultivated a habit that saw me sometimes wish bedtime happened earlier than 7pm because then my drinking time would start earlier.

I didn't view it as my 'drinking time' of course. It was 'me time'.

And, hello? I'm a busy mum, I deserve my 'me time'! I've had cancer for God's sake, this is my time to relax. *My* time.

And so, it began.

Working from home has been the making of me, professionally. I'm self-motivated, planful and ambitious and I've forged a respected and successful career as a blogger, freelancer writer and marketing consultant.

I work hard during the day but by 2pm, I'm itching to see my kids, cuddle them and find out about their day.

I miss them terribly during the week, but I love to work too, always have.

Evenings and weekends are my time to shut off from work and to enjoy time with my husband and kids.

I'm so lucky to work from home and arrange my hours to see them as much as possible. I attend most of their daycare and school functions and don't have to work in the evenings or on weekends 99% of the time.

I can't remember when it happened, and I'm filled with shame to admit this. But at some point that feeling of "I can't wait for my kids to get home" started to be followed not long after with "and when they are asleep, I can open the wine."

There. I said it. I haven't told many people that little gem. Shave my head and walk me down Shame Street.

I realise now that as much as I loved being with my children, there have been some distinct occasions when I wished time away.

I was actively thinking less about being in the moment with them and more about when I would get my next alcoholic drink.

My husband is the main car driver and so family lunches, dinners, parties and occasions could be a free for all for me if I wanted to have a drink.

We don't go out in the evenings often but on the rare chance of a date or girls' night out, I would go to town. I'd stay up until as late as possible and enjoy glasses of wine and fancy cocktails to relive a little of my past as a party girl.

My husband and I would talk frequently about how we needed to "cut back", "drink less", "be healthier".

I know now, of course, that him saying "we" really meant "me". I knew *I* was the one with the addiction.

Whilst he has always enjoyed a drink as much as I have, he can turn off the desire for one much easier. He also works out and has a physically active day job.

So, whilst my drinking has led me to pile on the kilos, or to at least be stunted from losing them, he didn't suffer physically from the effects of drinking.

That said, I can deal with the late nights and less sleep much better. I've been an insomniac since I was a teen and have become accustomed to surviving a day after very little sleep the night before. It isn't a skill I'm proud of.

I often wondered if drinking alcohol made my insomnia worse.

WebMD says alcohol and a good night's sleep don't mix:

"A new review of twenty-seven studies shows that alcohol does not improve sleep quality. According to the findings, alcohol does allow healthy people to fall asleep quicker and sleep more deeply for a while, but it reduces rapid eye movement (REM) sleep.

And the more you drink before bed, the more pronounced these effects. REM sleep happens about ninety minutes after we fall asleep. It's the stage of sleep when people dream, and it's thought to be restorative. Disruptions in REM sleep may cause daytime drowsiness, poor concentration, and rob you of needed ZZZs."

Source: https://www.webmd.com/sleep-disorders/news/20130118/alcohol-sleep

This makes sense to me as despite falling to sleep quickly when I was drunk, it didn't feel like good sleep and I was constantly waking. I put my light sleeping down to being a mum.

Drinking alcohol became useful to me, to help me sleep. I'd justified it. Of course, falling into a gentle sleep cannot compare to passing out after a downing a bottle of wine, I now know.

The side effects of drinking too much took their toll and over time, the hangovers I thought were forever gone returned.

If I had been drinking the night before, I would wake up exhausted, dehydrated, paranoid and irritable.

My tolerance for alcohol had increased over time and so whilst some women might not physically tolerate drinking a bottle of wine to themselves in one sitting, I could handle that. I'd been honing that particular skill for years.

But it was showing all over my face, physically. The tiredness, the sallow skin, the dark circles.

My work was suffering as I was foggy-headed and forgetful. Some of this is because of the side effects of chemo, but not all.

I gave up exercising. Too hard to do when you feel like shit.

My diet suffered. Late night sugary snacks pair up spectacularly with alcohol, no?

I couldn't remember the last time I had sex with my husband without having had a drink first.

Bloody hell. Bloody, bloody hell.

Three years ago, I was fearful I might die on the spot after being diagnosed with a shitty kind of cancer.

That I might not see my babies grow.

That I might not make my next birthday.

And here I was, shouting a big 'fuck off' to that and getting smashed every night out of the sheer habit of it.

Was drinking making me less fearful? Momentarily, until it wore off.

Was drinking making my cancer go away? Definitely not.

Was drinking making me forget the pain of the things wrong in my life? Well yes, for a short time only. But the pain came back and brought more painful pals with it.

And what about my liver? I mean, drinking so much surely must have had an effect by now?

But I couldn't cut down. I couldn't stop. I had tried and repeatedly failed.

It made me feel like a terrible person and certainly a God-awful mother. When the world and everyone I knew was shouting about 'living their best lives', here I was ruining mine from the inside out.

Not only that, but also hating myself for it. The guilt and anxiety were eating me up, and the shame pecked at me all day every day.

From the outside, I looked and acted like a functioning woman, mother and friend but on the inside, I was locked in a self-created hell with no key.

I was addicted to alcohol.

THE TURNING POINT

For months I had wanted to cut down but had only discussed this with my husband, GP and psychologist.

I'd even googled to find the local AA meeting but decided it wasn't for me.

As I firmly told my psychologist, "I don't want to be a teetotaller and quit altogether. I just want to cut back."

People do that all the time, don't they?

So many friends tell me how they've quit for a month or even three months.

For me, the only time I 100% quit drinking altogether was when I was pregnant and in the first few months of breastfeeding.

I didn't drink much during chemo but that was because I felt so shocking, rather than me purposefully abstaining.

On a night out with two girlfriends in early January 2019, I confessed about the amount I had been drinking to them.

One friend was shocked whilst the other, another mum of young kids, said she was drinking the same amount.

They both knew me as a big drinker and they both could drink a fair bit themselves although not to my 'standards' I would say.

Whilst the confession itself didn't get a massively negative reaction, saying it aloud seemed to make something change inside me.

I think it was the first time I said I was drinking too much, too often and I couldn't stop.

I was addicted to alcohol.

The night got messy, and we went to a bar until the early hours, dancing and chatting to locals.

We'd shared two bottles of wine between the three of us and two more drinks each, but I felt sober.

My tolerance levels had built up so much this large amount of alcohol had either barely affected me or was certainly taking far too long to take effect.

I've done a quick Google for some facts on alcohol tolerance and you know what came up at the top of the search results? Numerous posts on, 'How to increase your drinking tolerance'. Scary.

After a good scroll, I found the UK's Drinkaware site and their take on Tolerance is this:

"If you're drinking on a regular basis, then the amount of alcohol you need to get the same click or buzz gradually goes up," says Dr Nick Sheron, a liver specialist from Southampton University. So, if your brain has got used to a certain level of stimulation, you won't get that same 'buzz' if you drink less. Your tolerance can creep up without you even noticing. If you think your tolerance is rising, then think about whether you could be becoming dependent on alcohol. e.g. beginning to use it regularly to unwind after work, or to socialise."

Source: https://www.drinkaware.co.uk/advice/how-to-reduce-your-drinking/how-to-cut-down/how-to-take-a-break-and-reset-your-tolerance/

Looking around the bar, at my friends and other

revellers, I felt quite lonely. They were all having a much better time than me and I put it down to them being more relaxed. Because they were drunk.

Since a young age, I've been convinced drinking alcohol is a good way to relax.

So how did I deal with the awkwardness of feeling out of place? I drank more, and I drank it quickly.

I downed three or four vodka and sodas along with the group.

When it was May's turn to buy a round, she put a glass down in front of me and I immediately picked it up for a swig.

To my horror, it was water. Water? She was trying to 'water' me down.

Was I being a bad drunk? Was I showing myself up? Why did my best friend who apparently loved me want to put a damper on my night? Why kind of fuckery is this?

I asked her just that.

"Um, the water is mine," she said. "I want to slow down a bit, I feel a bit drunk."

Oh. Um. Oops.

The vodka finally kicked in and the night was fun and the next day the hangover left me feeling sorry for myself. I had that same old anxious and paranoid feeling of 'did something bad happen last night?'

This was two days after I vomited at the side of the road as my kids looked on. Two days.

You see, I was a real trooper when it came to drinking. I would power through hangovers, drink quickly to catch up to friends who had started before me and hit the hard stuff if it meant getting my buzz on sooner rather than later.

It's a skill one might add to their resume for a job as a professional partygoer.

But the alcohol I thought was relaxing me and helping me to melt away my fears only made them worse.

It's a depressant, you know.

"If you drink heavily and regularly, you're likely to develop some symptoms of depression. It's that good old brain chemistry at work again. Regular drinking lowers the levels of serotonin in your brain—a chemical that helps to regulate your mood.

Drinking heavily can also affect your relationships with your partner, family and friends. It can impact on your performance at work. These issues can also contribute to depression.

If you use drink to improve your mood or mask your depression, you may start a vicious cycle.

Warning signs alcohol is affecting your mood include:

Poor sleep after drinking

Feeling tired because of a hangover

Low mood

Experiencing anxiety in situations where you would normally feel comfortable."

Source: https://adf.org.au/drug-facts/alcohol/

In the cold light of day, I faced up to the fact I had a problem, and I needed help. I couldn't do it alone.

I decided at my next psychologist appointment I would make my problem with alcohol the only item on the agenda. She would help me find a solution to cut back and drink less.

At that point, cutting back was my only goal.

One *good* habit I had picked up in 2018 was to get back into reading. Well, audiobooks to be exact.

I've dived so deeply into it I'm ploughing through books on self-help for women in business at lightning speed and I'm loving it.

I searched for books about drinking and how to cut back and the results had one eye-catching option right at the top.

"How to Stop Drinking for Women" by Allen Carr.

Two things attracted me to the book. First, a heap of my friends had quit smoking with his "How to Quit Smoking" book over a decade ago.

Second, the title. The fact it addressed the reasons women in particular drink and how to help them stop. It spoke to me. Well, pretty obvious title, right?

The book debunks the theory you need 'willpower' to quit and I'll talk about willpower later.

Rather than trying to use willpower, Carr uncovered two of the reasons I was drinking so much. First, I discovered from an early age I've believed the hype that alcohol does something good for me, when it does not.

What started as a way to 'blend in' as a teen, be 'adult' in my twenties or 'relax' as a stressed-out mum has spiralled into the uncontrollable. But when we're all doing something, it's ok, right?

Carr took me back to my first alcoholic drink, well the one I first remember as a teenager when my sense of taste was fully developed. It was disgusting. As was my second, third and fourth.

But I kept going, practising if you like, because the

wanted outcome of blending in and feeling awesome completely overrode the revolting and poisonous taste. If only I could apply the same determination to doing more exercise or eating less chocolate. Something I'm working on, by the way.

If I could go back in time, I would tell teenage Mim off. "Look love, alcohol is gross. You've tried it, you hate it, stop now!" I would say to myself. "It isn't worth the expense, the ill-heath, the psychological damage and the hundreds of wasted hours it's stealing from you."

The second reason for my drinking, according to Carr, was I was addicted to alcohol. Plain and simple.

Reading this was like a lightbulb going on in my head. There I was with 'Addicted to Alcohol' label slapped on my forehead instantly. And weirdly, it made me feel good.

I felt relieved because it validated for me it wasn't my fault. I couldn't control my alcohol consumption. There was a reason it was controlling me. An addiction.

I knew from my circle of friends and family many addictions could also be resolved and cured. Therefore, mine could too.

It was liberating to know my situation had a cause, a label and a cure.

Cause – brainwashing.

Label – alcohol addiction.

Cure – oh, sweet baby Jesus, let this book be the cure.

And it was. I listened to the audiobook religiously every day for an hour here and there and, bit by bit, the 'brainwashing' was uncovered and reversed.

Hands up, it's what's led to me being so opinionated about why others drink. I'm convinced some others are also prey to society's brainwashed message of 'drinking alcohol is fun/helpful/necessary'.

Carr's book has simple and specific instructions to follow that made me feel safe with this knowledge. If I kept an open mind and followed his instructions, I would quit alcohol by the time I'd finished the book.

Not only would I quit, but it would be easy, without a dependence on willpower and I would no longer have any desire to drink alcohol anymore.

And, my friends, it worked. It really did.

It's a book I now recommend to anyone who has even a small interest in quitting drinking or even cutting back.

Before reading the book, I could not stop. I couldn't even cut down. I was addicted to drinking. But discovering that was a relief.

Learning it wasn't a 'willpower' thing took away all the feelings of inadequacy I had previously felt. I was addicted to drinking and I couldn't stop.

I wasn't weak, stupid or crazy, but alcohol was my addiction.

The Oxford Dictionary defines Alcoholism as:

"Addiction to the consumption of alcoholic drink; alcohol dependency."

The first part I can relate to. I was addicted to consuming alcohol. Most nights, wine.

It became something I would look forward to daily sitting down and having a drink because my day had been hard. Or amazing. Or sad. The best day ever. Or boring. Wine was the answer to all of life's unanswered questions.

The second part of that definition though, *dependent* on alcohol. I struggle with that. *Was I dependent on alcohol?*

I'm still learning, but I think I was.

More than anything, it was the *habit* of drinking.

7.00pm would roll around and after the kids were tucked up in bed, the routine of Netflix/snacks/wine would begin. Most nights. Some weeks, every night.

Which may sound familiar to many of you. And for most people, that might not be an issue. For me, it was.

Because when it came to the thought of cutting back, I just couldn't.

I listened to the book every day for a couple of weeks and from the first chapter I was hooked as I discovered my issue wasn't my fault.

I *was* addicted to alcohol.

It gave me answers and started to unravel the brainwashing about drinking I had been subjected to for over twenty years.

You don't have to stop drinking whilst you're reading the book. In fact, it's encouraged you carry on as normal, if you want to. Until the moment you have your last drink.

I had my last alcoholic drink the day before I finished the book. It took me about two weeks to read it because busy mum, etc.

I didn't tell anyone I was reading the book or preparing to quit drinking. In January in Australia, businesses shut down for some time and my next appointment with my psychologist wasn't until early February.

So, I told no one.

Until I finished the book. Then I told my husband.

"I've quit alcohol," I said, casually on January 23rd,

2019. "I had my last drink yesterday."

"No, you haven't," he said. "And we have loads of wine in the fridge."

I'll be honest, this had crossed my mind too as I was reading the book. What a waste! Although that wine was cheap as chips special offer stuff so as much as it pained me to waste the money, it demonstrated I wasn't particular when I purchased it.

I could afford to let it go, in every way.

"I don't care," I said. "I've stopped drinking forever and I would appreciate it if you could please stop too, at least for now whilst I'm adjusting."

That last bit was met with a glare. But he knew how much I had been struggling. I had no other answers for my issue with drinking. He had no answers. He was willing to put his faith in this as a possible solution.

Reading the book has one major impact. It takes away any *desire* to drink alcohol. I was not inclined to put alcohol into my body and suffer its effects anymore.

That was the easy part, not craving alcohol.

One mountain I still had to climb was overcoming the *habit* of drinking.

The "it's 7pm, the kids are in bed, let's crack open the wine and watch Netflix!" habit.

The habit of having a drink after a hard day. Or a not-hard day.

The habit of drinking at home because we have kids and can't go out. Or we can't afford to go out and drinking at home is cheaper.

Because I'd just bought lovely new wine glasses and what else was I going to put in them.

The habit was just as much of a challenge to overcome as the urge to drink alcohol.

What is a Habit? James Clear, author of one of my favourite books, "Atomic Habits", says:

"Habits are the small decisions you make and actions you perform every day. According to researchers at Duke University, habits account for about forty percent of our behaviours on any given day. Your life today is essentially the sum of your habits. How in shape or out of shape you are? A result of your habits. How happy or unhappy you are? A result of your habits. How successful or unsuccessful you are? A result of your habits.

What you repeatedly do (i.e. what you spend time thinking about and doing each day), ultimately forms the person you are, the things you believe, and the personality that you portray."

Source: https://jamesclear.com/habits

I'm quite the fan of routines and they've served me well for many years at work, home and getting stuff done as a busy mum.

I thrive on the results of the good habits I've set. It means I often instinctively do the right thing without questioning it.

But there are some bad habits in my life I have yet to overcome and drinking too much alcohol too frequently was my worst.

It topped the list of my 'most hated things about myself' list.

It came first in my personal "So you think you can drink?" reality show style drink-off. I always invited it back the next week.

I was really, really good at drinking.

Breaking the habit was bolstered by Allen Carr's book.

Taking away the desire to want to drink alcohol meant I was 95% there with kicking my addiction to alcohol.

That remaining 5% would be an ongoing struggle for a while and I think for the rest of my life to some extent.

But I was about to embark on a new life. A life without alcohol. One with more control.

That wasn't to say I wasn't nervous about the change and if my new alcohol-free existence might transpire to become a mundane, sombre affair.

Would I be boring? Would my confidence wane? Could I still be around people who were drinking? Would I still enjoy... karaoke?

I was feeling apprehensive yet brave. I'll come back to the fears I had later in the book and let you know if they have become my reality and, if so, how I'm dealing with them.

Let me tell you how, after reading Carr's book, I broke the habit of drinking alcohol.

BREAKING MY HABIT DAY BY DAY

I planned as much as possible. To plan for success in conquering my alcoholic demons. Super Mim would forge a steadfast plan to eradicate the grape-flavoured baddies and save her liver from uncertain death.

Here's a timeline from days one to 100. The first couple of nights were easy peasy.

Day 1 - January 23rd, 2019

I planned an early night so as soon as the kids were in bed and settled, off I went to bed myself.

I smugly tucked myself in for the night, content my non-drinking future had got off to a smashing start.

Could I get to sleep? Not a chance.

My mind raced, not with the urge to drink, but many other real-life thoughts that by this time on an average evening I would have quashed down with my first chug of wine.

Had my day been good? Was I productive enough? Could I have done more?

What did I need to do tomorrow? Would I meet that deadline?

Why was my To-do list so long? How are we going to pay the bills this month? And next?

Why didn't I stick to my diet today? What can I do to

stick to it tomorrow?

I'm not tired. Why am I not I tired? I feel sort of tired. Why can't I sleep? WTF can't I get to sleep?

I was stressed already, and it was only 7.30pm but those feelings plus friends rotated around my head for hours until way after midnight.

I could have got up and watched TV or read a book and in hindsight I should have done the latter, something to distract me. But I was anxious I didn't want to put myself in the physical position where I might drink.

The next morning, instead of waking up feeling bright-eyed and bushy-tailed, I felt shattered and a bit deflated but also still resolute I am no longer a drinker. But I continued to keep a diary each day of how I was tracking with sobriety.

Day 2 - January 24th, 2019

Despite the little sleep from the night before, I have the sense of 'elation' Allen Carr talks about in the book. He asks readers to make themselves feel elated, even if they don't yet feel it. I remember feeling weird about it originally but now it comes much more naturally.

It isn't that I feel elated about not drinking alcohol, it's all the things I will gain by not drinking.

At work, my day is the same as usual, no better or worse than previous days.

But, you see, the daytime was never my issue. I was never that roll-out-of-bed-and-grab-the-vodka-addicted-to-alcohol-girl.

It's the 7pm thing that was the problem. And the immediate run up to that.

With one day of sobriety under my belt, I decide it's time to tell the world about my new alcohol-free lifestyle. Because I'm an over-sharer these days, it seems.

I open Instagram and record a series of videos about my decision to quit alcohol. I nervously giggle through my reasons for giving up the grog and how I've done it. I'm inundated with messages of support and questions. More on that later.

3.30pm rolls along and I wind down work and think about what's for dinner. The hubs is getting the kids from school and they'll be home in less than an hour. And this is the time the old habit rears its head again.

My old routine:

    3.30pm: stop work

    4.00pm: make dinner

    4.30pm: hang out with kids

    6.45pm: start the bedtime routine

    7.00pm: Wine! Wine! Wine! Wine! Wine!

    Sometime later: bed

Told you I loved routine. And this had been the routine for most nights for as long as I can remember.

Oh, but I like occasional spontaneity, don't get me wrong. On 'I'm on a diet' days, it might be vodka, lime and soda.

That night I spend a few hours googling and reading about the side effects of long-term drinking and how long it would take for alcohol to leave my body.

Most literature I find didn't address the circumstances of someone in my position but rather people who have abused alcohol for many years in much larger quantities than me.

The side effects talked about the shakes or 'DTs'.

WebMD addresses what causes withdrawal symptoms:

"Alcohol has what doctors call a depressive effect on your system. It slows down brain function and changes the way your nerves send messages back and forth.

Over time, your central nervous system adjusts to having alcohol around all the time. Your body works hard to keep your brain in a more awake state and to keep your nerves talking to one another.

When the alcohol level suddenly drops, your brain stays in this keyed-up state. That's what causes withdrawal."

They listed many possible physical withdrawals from alcohol symptoms on WebMD including:

- Anxiety
- Shaky hands
- Headache
- Nausea
- Vomiting
- Insomnia
- Sweating
- Confusion
- Racing heart
- High blood pressure
- Fever
- Heavy sweating

Source: https://www.webmd.com/mental-health/addiction/alcohol-withdrawal-symptoms-treatments#1

I hadn't experienced any of these so far and I wondered if I would. Was I *that* much of a drinker that I might?

Being the paranoid person I am since having cancer, I put myself under an imaginary microscope and started to question every ache, pain and sniff of a shudder. Eventually I fall asleep.

Day 3 - January 25th, 2019

It's Friday night and I'm... sitting on the sofa and watching Netflix... with a glass of... water! Amazing! I'm making this non-drinking thing really happen.

Thing is, drinking water by day is *healthy* but drinking water at night is *boring,* isn't it? So boring. Feels wrong, feels like 'What's the point?'

So, I simultaneously watch Riverdale and play games on my iPhone at the same time. I recall a quote about idle hands and devils.

An observation, despite the attempt at multi-tasking, I'm really *watching* the TV show. And taking it in.

I think about all the times I've had to re-watch whole episodes of TV shows the next day because I couldn't recall a thing that happened when I watched drunk. *Have you done that too? You have, haven't you?*

Three episodes in and I'm done. It isn't even 10.30pm and I'm shattered. In the olden days of last week, I rarely got to bed before 11pm, often way after midnight.

I look at turning in 'early' as a treat to myself and I need to catch up on sleep from losing it the previous night.

Off to bed I went and fell asleep just before midnight.

Day 4 - January 26th, 2019

Well, I cannot recall the last Saturday morning I didn't feel some effects of having drunk alcohol the night before. It feels good today to feel like this.

Today will be my first social test and I'm ready to face it. We're celebrating a family member's birthday.

The hubs had three glasses. Wow! People do get louder with every drink, right?

"Am I judging them?" I think to myself. I mean, as much as I know I was a 'happy drunk', I can also remember me and my friends getting louder as the night went on when we drank. Some mornings, my throat would be sore from the back and forth shouting in bars. Or on sofas at their house or mine.

I wonder if this is what I'm in for now, becoming annoyed as other people drink and get loud while I sit quietly fuming a little.

After we get home and the kids are in bed, it's another Netflix night. I should warn you since our kids are little, we don't go out much in the evening. One reason I justified drinking so much at home. Every night was an 'indoor date night'.

I turn in again at around 10pm, a bit deflated at how boring sitting in front of Netflix feels. I'm trying to cut down my intake of carbs and sugar at the same time as going sober and it's sapping the joy out of me a bit. I consider being kinder to myself with the food limitations because I'm worried if I restrict myself too much, I'll binge on the empty calories in alcohol as I have in the past.

Sleep comes a little easier but we're having an issue now with one or both kids waking up in the middle of the night and getting into our bed.

It's fine when it's one of them but our queen won't take a family of four and these kids kick and sprawl.

The hubs kindly escorts them back to their rooms most nights but tonight I find it difficult to get back to sleep.

I download an app called… wait for it… 'I am Sober'. I love goal setting and tracking, and this will be an easy way for me to see how far I've come. Plus, I set up a daily reminder to keep me motivated.

Source: https://iamsober.com/

Day 5 - January 27th, 2019

Another weekend morning with no hangover. I've got this! After some frantic middle-of-the-night googling I also conclude I'm unlikely to get any of the withdrawal symptoms I'd read about. I feel like they would have started by now so perhaps I've escaped them.

I try to not let my mind wonder if that meant I didn't have a drinking problem after all. I don't want to give myself any excuses to fall off this wagon.

I tell myself firmly that "alcohol does absolutely nothing for me" and go about my day.

Tonight, I'm having a very early night because tomorrow, I've decided I'm a 5am person.

I've wanted to be a 5am person for a while. You know, the women who get up at 5am to go jogging. Or get the housework done or read a book before the kids wake up. Or do a bunch of productive stuff that non-5am people don't have the time to do.

I set my alarm for 5am, chuffed with myself that as well as being a super-healthy non-drinker, I am also now a 5am person. I am kicking all the goals lately. I LOVE the new me. Na-night.

Day 6 - January 28th, 2019

Alarm goes off at 5am and fuck that.

I mean, I'm comfortable, warm and tired. I have no actual appointment to get up at 5am for so why the hell would I? I do not. I reset the alarm until 7am.

It was worth a go. Let's kick that goal another day. Not today.

During the day my phone buzzes with a reminder from Timehop of the Australia Day celebrations we used to attend, years ago. These reminders are always a day or so late on Timehop.

Images of me and my friends with temporary tattoos of Australian flags on our chests, clutching pints of cider and wrapping our arms around each other from midday to midnight.

I won't pretend they weren't fun times because they were. But booze aside, I no longer feel the pull of that stuff. Family BBQs, trips to the local park or swimming pool with the kids are more my things now on those kinds of days.

As I've got older, I still love to go out with friends, but the crowds affect me. I have no interest in queuing to get in anywhere, being elbowed at a bar, someone accidentally spilling their drink on me or paying over the odds for a cheap glass of wine.

And don't get me started on bars that don't have enough seats for anyone! Jesus, I *am* forty.

So, looking at these pictures doesn't make me miss the booze one bit.

Days 7-10 - January 29th - February 1st, 2019

This week has been busy with work and the days have blended together somewhat. School and day care started back and many of our daytime and evening routines have recommenced.

School drop offs, pickups, lunches, laundry, form-filling and packing bags keeps my mind occupied a lot of the time.

A work trip proves insightful as two of the girls share they have also quit drinking for similar reasons to me. I'm over the moon. It feels like a movement!

Why can't everyone in the world just stop and make alcohol unavailable and then I will stop getting twitchy from 7.00pm onwards every night?

The 7.00pm wine twitch is still real. And now I'm obsessing over thinking about wine. And how I'm thinking about thinking about wine. So much thinking.

One girl recommended another book about sobriety called "The Unexpected Joys of Being Sober" by Catherine Gray. I've downloaded the audiobook and one paragraph in, I'm already hooked.

This girl is talking to my soul. I mean, she's literally speaking to me as she narrates the audiobook and I think I might have fallen in love with her a little.

Someone else gets it.

Whilst Catherine's story gets more extreme than mine, I relate to so much of what she says and highly recommend it.

A friend, Eva, shared with me a few days ago I've inspired her to quit drinking too and she's picked up the Allen Carr book. It's going well! Eva said:

"I'm feeling really empowered not drinking. It's a funny feeling. The book is great so far, so many things have stuck in my head. I've still got a lot of the book to read but I've read the first three and a half chapters and love it. Thanks so much for the recommendation."

That's how I feel too: empowered. In control. Finally.

Day 11

Saturday rolls round again. A friend invites me out tonight and this would be my first night out since being sober.

But I'm shattered from the insomnia, I have random neck pain and I'm not in the mood.

After a shower and getting dressed, I sit at my computer intending to tick something off tomorrow's To-do list.

Instead, I am inclined to write. I write a blog post, announcing to the world, or my tiny corner of the internet, I am sober. I pour my heart out, just a little, about why I've made the decision and how I'm doing it.

I contemplate it being a bad idea to show my demons so publicly. So few friends and family know about my issues with drinking and I wonder if this is the way to communicate it. Will they understand?

Will I be judged? By the people I know or strangers? What about trolls?

My gut tells me to hit Publish, and it's gone, released to the world. I feel relieved. Like I've taken another step to healing.

I share my fears with Eva, who is now sharing her non-drinking journey with me too. She helps me focus on the positive and tells me, "By sharing your experience, you're helping others."

The thought of an early night, or at least a quiet night in, is so much more appealing than going out with my friend and I turn down the invite of a night out.

I decide rather than have avoided confronting my demons, this is a win. You see, in the olden days (I'll keep calling them that by the way), I wouldn't have cared about being tired, or the neck pain, or even the company *that* much. If a night out was on offer, the alcohol alone was enough to pull me aboard the Good Ship Shit-faced.

So, I'm quietly rejoicing that I felt no pull to drink and no disappointment in not being able to.

Is this getting easier?

Day 12

The hubs promised me a lie in today, to rest my sore neck and catch up on some sleep.

He's taken the kids to swimming lessons and I get up at around 8am. My neck isn't too bad, and I feel quite… alive today.

Again, I sit at my desk to write and the thought crosses my mind I might write a book. As you do.

I recall a time, about seven years earlier when I'd gone back to the UK to visit family and friends. I was in the back of Marie's car as she drove us through the picturesque Derbyshire countryside with her beautiful Irish mum, Orla, in the front passenger seat.

I gleefully recanted tales of life in Australia and even stories of our school days, growing up together and the fun we'd had. Both laughed along with me and I was on cloud nine. Telling stories has always been a love of mine

– hooking people in, making them smile, laugh and cry.

"You've a book in you, Mim!" Orla said.

And my heart raced because it was something I hadn't given any thought to in decades.

I mean, I write for a living, but it isn't the same.

During my school years, I knew there *was* a book in me. Many books. I suppose I had a sense of arrogance many young writers have and patiently waited until the book idea *came* to me. It did not come to me. It just didn't.

My inspiration for telling stories in a book faded over time and I suppose my confidence in even contemplating the possibility did too.

But in the back of my mind, somewhere hidden away, the longing to write a book of my own never left me.

This is not the book I intended to write. Not by a long shot.

But here I am, at my computer, tapping away into Microsoft Word and writing a book. Where will it lead? Will I give up after the first day? Will it be something I lose passion for or forget about again? I wrote 8283 words in that first writing session.

"Pretty sure writing a book isn't that easy!" I joked to myself when the kids came home, and I shut the computer down.

Day 13

Last night I had the worst insomnia for a while, not getting to sleep until past 2am.

I'm tired and disappointed but that sense of elation is still here. And *confidence.*

I know even though I've only had a few hours' sleep, I can *do* today because I wasn't drinking alcohol last night. And I haven't drunk in almost two weeks.

Work is busy and my list of stuff to do is long, but I go through the motions of getting shit done.

All day though, I'm itching to get back to the book. The words I need to get onto paper are swirling around my head, pining to be released. But it's exciting and I haven't felt this surge in a long time.

I wonder if the passion is coming from my newfound energy or the topic itself. The elation and positivity I'm feeling about being sober is something I can't contain, and I want to share it with the world. I want to tell everyone I meet how amazing my life without alcohol will be and how they too can benefit from the unexpected joys of being sober. (Catherine Gray, I love your phrase so much.)

Whether it's the passion for the topic or clarity my mind now has every day, I embrace the surge and resume writing. Up to 11,000 words now. How long are books, anyway?

I google "How many words does a book have?" Google provides many answers that don't really help, and I realise I'm distracted and shut that down.

Day 16

Still struggling at 7pm. Where is The Fun? I think The Fun has gone.

If you read this, please send The Fun.

I keep a daily gratitude list to bring on the positive vibes. The things I'm most grateful for, the good stuff. Like my kids, our good health, the ability to do a job I love.

Chocolate. Sobriety.

Day 19

The Fun was not sent and instead I have a sore throat and a cold.

Is it toxins leaving my body?

Every time I feel a twinge, ache or physical symptom, I wonder if it's alcohol related. Which is a nice change from assuming it's cancer related.

I have a read of Catherine Gray's blog and discover something shocking. More so for me than her. Something I missed whilst reading her book.

"I have been sober since September 2013. Before that date, I had worked my way up to an average of seven bottles of wine a week, or 70 units, a life-endangering amount of alcohol. I was only taking one or two days off from drinking a week. Yet, very few people around me, aside from immediate family and my best friend, knew I was addicted."

Reading Catherine's book, the situations drinking got her into and the physical alcohol-related symptoms she felt during her drinking years and throughout withdrawal shocked me.

But now reading this statement on her blog, what scared me the most is we were drinking the same amount.

Why hadn't I been affected as much physically? Or have I, and I don't know it yet?

Day 20

It might be having a temperature, but I dream about

absentmindedly having a sip of wine on a night out and in the dream, I instantly have the world's worst hangover. I'm parched, hot and ill.

It's the last dream I have before I wake up and when I do, I feel ill. But it's from the cold of course, not the imaginary hangover.

Alcohol is haunting my dreams. Or is daydreaming about alcohol following me into my dreams?

Day 21

Three weeks in and 'Yay!' to me. I'm still feeling elated and I'm so proud of myself.

But this gratitude list thing is hard to do. Kids and health. Kids and health. I can't say that every day though, can I?

I reflect on the opposite, the negative thoughts that come into my mind I don't push away. I'm working with my psychologist to give less power to them and I've developed a personal strategy about this. When I think the bad thoughts, there are three options available to them:

Fuck It: there are some things I can't change or don't count. Such as 'what if my cancer comes back?'

I have very little control over that happening and there is no point in wasting time thinking about that before it happens. It's wasting time and getting me down. So, I acknowledge them and then push those kinds of thoughts away.

File It: these are the things I need to address, but not right away. I can't worry about all the things all the time.

Feel It: the hardest one, sitting with those uncomfortable emotions. The kind where there's no point in denying the thought exists or that the scary feeling isn't real.

I'm so happy to hear from Eva and how well she's finding being AF is going for her:

"Sobriety frigging rocks! I'm seventeen days without a drink and it's hand down one of the best decisions I've made, and I've really surprised myself."

I couldn't agree more with this because I'm surprising myself every day too. It's amusing to wonder how on earth I've quit alcohol altogether when weeks ago I was struggling to go a single night without it.

Day 22

I'm still blown away by how many emails and messages I'm getting from my blog readers who have been inspired to quit alcohol for similar reasons to me.

'S' messaged me after I posted on Facebook:

"Thanks so much for this. I'm in the same place and I don't know where to start. It's all so scary."

I remember how scared I felt too, the feeling of being controlled and not being able to escape. It was terrifying. To have gone from being so scared to so empowered in twenty-two days blows my mind. I'm excited for S too.

Day 30 & 31

We went away this weekend with friends who we would have, in the past, drank heavily with.

It was a fun weekend, but it brought some cravings for alcohol, being surrounded by so many bottles of wine and cider.

That said, I don't feel like our experience of the holiday suffered in a negative way at all. In fact, I slept like a baby and loved waking up feeling so refreshed each day.

Day 41

The days and nights are getting easier and I'm feeling stronger and more resolute by the day.

But one thing has surprised me quite a lot. Weight gain.

Given the number of empty calories I'd been consuming during my drinking days, I expected the weight to fall off me but it's creeping on. A few kilos now.

So, as much as I'm feeling proud of myself, the weight gain is having a less than positive impact on my mindset.

I get it somewhat. I mean, I have been upping the sugar and carb snacks as a bit of crutch to take my mind off alcohol. But it's time to change that and I start today with that goal; to make healthier decisions about food.

Day 48

Not one to do things by halves, I jump on the plant-based bandwagon.

Over the years, I've read a lot about the health benefits of eating a plant-based diet and not consuming meat and dairy. Today I go cold turkey on eating animals.

Day 49

I'm seven weeks alcohol-free and it feels amazing!

The biggest change physically is the sleep. So much sleep. I'm occasionally still having issues in getting to sleep but once I'm out, I'm out all night. Having blamed being a mum for my light sleeping for so many years, this feels like a mini miracle.

Was my alcohol consumption the real problem?

The next-day anxiety after a night on the wine is a thing of the past too and it's making me feel so much more in control and less stressed. I feel wonderful.

Day 60

This is now the longest time I've been without drinking alcohol except for my pregnancies and when I was going through chemo.

I'm still asked why I've made this a permanent change, rather than cutting back and I explain repeatedly why. I don't mind this; I feel like opening the conversation can only be a positive thing for others to understand my decision and act themselves if they need and want to.

It's getting easier and I'm resigned to never drinking again but occasionally, I wonder if I might drink again. At a wedding, or New Year, or something like that.

But as much as it's only been sixty days, I still feel strongly I'll never be a 'one glass of wine' girl. I would drink to get drunk. Not falling over shit-faced drunk, but I want that feeling of being relaxed and getting a buzz.

And, for me, that isn't healthy. Because I was blurring my life away. I purposefully drank to 'forget' or to 'minimise' the shit storm around me.

Alcohol was numbing the pain but fuelling the anxiety fire and I appreciate now I was only masking my demons, not facing them.

Now I must face them head on, stone cold sober. It's

scary. But I understand I need to face them, as tough as it sometimes is.

So, my plan is still to be sober forever. And it's exciting because the health benefits of quitting alcohol I'm already feeling are amazing.

I'll talk more about those later.

Day 64

I've come to Sydney for the weekend and been out for dinner with three girlfriends. They share a bottle of wine and it doesn't bother me at all. In fact, I'm growing quite the fan of kombucha, smoothies and juices and they're feeling like a real treat.

After a fun-filled night with so much chat and laughing, we head back to my friend's house where I'm staying.

All is going well until I stumble down the steps in her garden in the dark and land awkwardly.

I can feel and hear the cracks, snaps and pops on the way to the ground and I know something is very, very wrong.

For a few minutes I'm shaking but can't move and upon standing up I realise the extent of the injuries to both feet isn't good and we head to Emergency.

I'm asked three times by the nurses and doctors how much I've had to drink. *Really?*

I mean, I get that I'm chatty and it's 11.30pm but I haven't drunk and I'm not displaying any signs of being drunk.

After an x-ray, the doctor tells me there's nothing wrong except for a sprain and we head back to my friends although, I know this level of pain goes beyond sprains; particularly in my left foot. (I find out later they misdiagnosed my condition and I had three metatarsal fractures. Grr).

Day 75

Today we're off to a wedding, a friend of my husbands. I'm still in a lot of pain from the accident but looking forward to socialising and getting outside with the kids.

The wedding, which is outside, is a beautiful ceremony, and the bride looks amazing.

I get into a conversation with two guests about giving up alcohol and explaining why I'm drinking water.

They tell me, whilst clutching a bottle of beer each, that they 'don't drink' either. Um, ok.

I get this a lot. People leaping to justify why they're drinking or how much they usually drink when I haven't even asked them. It's weird but I shrug it off.

Day 77

Eleven weeks alcohol-free. Eleven weeks! I still can't quite believe how far I've come and pinch myself at such a massive achievement.

It's still so hard though. I still think how 'nice' it would be to crack open a bottle of wine with the hubs.

But the reason for wanting the wine, the dependency and the addiction, is still there.

It makes me feel sad because I thought by now, I wouldn't feel like this, as occasional as it is.

But, as much as I still think about going back to old

ways, I haven't, and I won't. And I'm still very proud of myself.

In these moments, when I have pangs for wine, they solidify for me I made the right decision.

I'm not craving wine. I'm craving escape. And that's the unhealthy part.

I'm continuing to work on facing my fears instead of ignoring them and I've started to read a brilliant book by Brené Brown called 'Rising Strong'. It's helping me to see how my fears are here to help me grow further and success beyond them.

Day 84

I'm now twelve weeks into my new alcohol-free life and five weeks into plant-based living. I'm feeling great!

These numbers, the days and weeks, they motivate me to keep going.

I imagine adding zeros on to the end of them and know if I'm feeling this good now, it will get so much better yet by then.

Day 90

Today I watched "The Call to Courage" by Brené Brown on Netflix and wow, what a revelation it has been.

I realise since my cancer diagnosis; I have been living in fear and allowing that fear to paralyse me.

Whilst a certain level of cautiousness is normal and rational, I've been letting it consume me instead of living a full happy life.

I've been paranoid feeling happiness will jinx me. I get

that now. And I think the alcohol was keeping me in this bubble where I thought I was self-medicating, but I was perpetuating the problem, not solving it.

I want to be brave and courageous. I want to get in the arena too. And one day, I want to meet Brené Brown and thank her for empowering me.

Day 100

I passed the 100 days mark!

Last night, I dreamed I was at an event with the hubs and some friends and he was drinking red wine. I was so disappointed in my dream.

Then, I looked down at the glass I was holding, and it was also red wine. I felt sick because I'd blown it and my reaction was to down the whole glass.

Of course, then I felt worse: guilt, failure, inadequacy, shame, anger.

All the feelings I had each morning after I had tried to stop drinking the night before and failed.

But it was just a dream. I didn't drink. I didn't fail.

I have nothing to feel guilty about and I'm so proud I'm winning the fight against one of my biggest battles.

Telling others about my alcohol addiction was tough but enlightening and led me to learn a lot about their own relationship with alcohol as much as my own.

THE REACTION FROM FAMILY AND FRIENDS

Telling my husband had been the first step, and I contemplated keeping my decision to quit alcohol to just the two of us and my doctors.

My husband had known I had a problem already. He spends time with me every evening. He knew how much I was drinking; he was drinking a lot with me. So, we both had a bit of an issue together.

I hesitated before telling my family, friends and blog readers before I did. First, well, it's a bit private and a lot embarrassing.

Second, I think I've developed a bit of a rep as a 'quitter' to my friends. Not in the good sense.

It's mainly diet-related because I've done all the diets. Each time, I've been so excited and motivated about the big, positive changes I'm going to make I've shouted it from the rooftops. I've wanted to bring everyone along for the ride to good health and smaller jeans. But inevitably, I've quit each time and felt ashamed when people ask, "How's the diet going?" and I've had to reply solemnly, "It's not."

I can't decide if it's rude for them to ask or if me proactively pulling them into the conversation in the first place has given them permission to make comments and judgements. I think it comes down to them showing concern and me self-judging.

However, I decided early on I *would* share my decision with everyone. And in fact, talking about being addicted became my new go-to conversation.

I shared my story on my blog and social channels, with family, friends and colleagues. Everyone.

I've quit drinking alcohol.

When a conversation started up with, well, anyone, it went a bit like this:

Them: "Hey Mim, how are you?"

Me: "Really good thanks, I quit alcohol."

Cue intense look from them.

Or

Them: "Hi Mim, how are you tracking on that project?"

Me: "It's going well and also I quit drinking wine."

Them: "Um, ok."

It didn't matter the conversation's topic, who was asking or why, I quickly turned the conversation to how I'd divorced alcohol. And it was therapeutic to share. For me, anyway.

And the reactions surprised me—a lot more than I expected them to.

"How long have you been drinking too much?"

The first friend asked me how long I'd been drinking so much, and I heard myself saying, "About three months, maybe six."

My husband raised an eyebrow, and that pissed me off. I wasn't lying.

But then it dawned on me a few days later when I recall a conversation I'd had with a nurse at my doctor's surgery. I had told her I was drinking 1-1.5 bottles of wine a night a few times a week.

That was over a year ago. Fuck. I wasn't lying, I'd forgotten I suppose. Blocked it out. Or blacked it out. Every hungover day blurring into the next until poof, a year of heavy drinking passes by.

"But you don't have a problem with drinking!"

There were some reactions from friends, family and acquaintances I wasn't expecting. I mean, everyone has been supportive for sure and most people have been surprised and didn't even realise I had a problem.

That gives me mixed feelings. Did I hide it that well? Was my problem not as big as I thought it was?

Niamh, one of my oldest friends in the UK said:

"I didn't even realise you had a problem, and I was quite surprised. I was almost in denial for you as it seemed to come out of the blue. (I'm sure it didn't of course.) I thought it was quite a drastic move at first but as we live at opposite sides of the planet, I hadn't seen how alcohol has affected you since having kids. I understand the lure of having a glass of wine when the kids are in bed. And how quickly that can turn to two. It's made me rethink my attitude to drinking and to question myself too."

My close friend, Sara, was equally surprised:

"You aren't the typical picture I had in my head of someone who has a drinking problem. I knew you liked to drink and that you probably drank more than me, but it never crossed my mind that it was an issue for you. At first, I thought you were overreacting but the more you have talked about it and explained it, and maybe even gained clarity on it yourself, it has helped me to understand also."

"Why don't you just cut down?"

Many people have questioned why I stopped altogether rather than just cut down, but it wasn't a possibility for me, I soon found.

Plus, as Allen Carr said, "it takes immense willpower to cut down because the tendency with all addictive drugs is to take more. You're constantly fighting the urge to have another fix. Eventually, the addict cracks and ends up taking even more of the drug than they were in the first place. Cutting down makes a drug seem more precious, not less. That's how addiction works."

After I confided more about the reasons I needed to quit, they understood.

"Something needed to happen whether it was working hard on drinking in moderation or going straight to cold turkey," said Damian.

When people suggest I cut down instead of quitting, my response is always the same:

I want to stop because of the health implications drinking that much was having on me. The fact it was masking different problems I had and how addicted to alcohol I had become.

It was costing me in many ways such as spending quality time with my kids and my husband and the negative health implications. It was costing me the next day in the anxiety I felt about having drunk so much again and how I was beating myself up. And financially, the amount we were spending on alcohol, particularly wine, even though it was cheap wine, was ridiculous. So, it was a financial cost to us too.

Some might think I'm weak or I don't have the willpower to cut down. Or I'm not trying hard enough.

But none of those things are true. I now realise I was addicted to alcohol, and that's the reason I couldn't stop. It wasn't my fault. I tried, trust me, I tried.

Allen Carr strongly believes using 'willpower' won't assist in quitting any addiction because of the sheer effort it takes to constantly apply it.

"It's the people who use the 'willpower method' who find it hard. The 'willpower method' refers to any other method of treating drug addiction that leaves the addict believing they're sacrificing some pleasure or crutch and they therefore have to apply willpower every day for the rest of their lives to fight the urge to take the drug."

And this makes so much sense to me because I can apply to every other addiction and obsession in my life that I've tried to cut back on. The more I think about not being allowed to eat something, see someone, do something, well, the more I want to.

With alcohol, I concluded it wasn't adding anything positive to my life. And that's one of the main messages in Allen Carr's book. He undid the brainwashing that had me convinced of the opposite.

Now I know alcohol does nothing good for me.

When I started reading his book, I had fought against this. I told myself drinking alcohol *was* adding to my life, enhancing it, helping me to be *me*.

Drinking alcohol was social and enjoyable. I enjoyed the taste. It helped me relax.

But I now realise alcohol wasn't giving me any of the benefits I perceived it did. It really wasn't.

"Why do you need to quit forever?"

I get asked this all the time. Why don't I cut down for a month or three months and then when I drink again, I'll have a better grip of it, and I won't be as bad?

And yes, I went into this process thinking that might be the case, but it isn't going to be the case for me. I don't intend to ever drink alcohol again.

I think if I was to resume drinking, I would eventually get addicted to it again. And I've never been a "one glass of wine" girl anyway.

And I've never had any interest in having a slight buzz of alcohol or drinking for the 'taste of a lovely glass of wine'. That has never been me. I always drank to get drunk, whether it's a slight buzz to take the edge of the day off. Or because I'm going on a big night out and I want the confidence to dance on the dance floor in front of everyone.

Or I'm going to a party with people I don't know, and I want the confidence to relax.

So, I've never been interested in only one glass and the chances of me ever being that person is slim to none.

Plus, I'd believe the hype again that alcohol was adding something good to my life when I know it isn't.

"You won't stick with it, you'll quit!"

A handful of people doubted me in the beginning and said, "Oh, you won't stick at this." They mean it in a jovial way and that's the manner I've taken it as well because I am not very good at quitting things or starting healthy lifestyle habits.

I appreciate I've got a track record of announcing to the world I'm taking on a new health regime or exercise plan and then not following through.

So, I understand why people who love me and who know me would have assumed I wouldn't follow through with this. But at this point, they realise I'm serious and they have a better understanding of why.

Since quitting, I've continued to be as social as I was before. I've stayed up late, chatted and laughed with friends. I've had five-hour long karaoke sessions and weekends away and proven to them, and to myself, I'm still the same social Mim I was before.

I'm just as chatty and just as loud, but hopefully less obnoxious and a lot more mindful.

I don't miss the next-day anxiety of, "Did I drink too much and was I a dickhead?"

"Well, I don't have a problem."

One thing that takes me back a little is when people ask me how *much* I used to drink. I'm certain I've never asked anyone once how much *they* drink. Yet it's the first thing many ask me when I tell them I've quit.

I've been loath to share the amount I drank until now. I worry the amount will either horrify them or they'll use it to justify the amount they're drinking and potentially deny their own problem.

I've found there's a lot of denial, though I haven't voiced it with anyone.

But at least half of the people I've told have said something like, "Oh, well I have a complete grip on my alcohol consumption." Or "I know when to cut down." Or "I can stop whenever I want to, but I know that I can drink just one glass a day or one glass every now and again."

It comes across to me like, "I'm fine, *I* don't have a problem." Which sometimes makes me wonder, are you sure? Because you seem defensive. And I hope you don't.

I think people are quick to forget or deny how much *they* really drink because they're focusing on my alcohol consumption and trying hard to justify their own.

It's another reason I'm sharing my story because rather than get on my soapbox and point the finger at others. I hope it might inspire other mums to consider making changes too if they feel the need.

But really, when you tell me you don't share *my* issue, when I didn't even ask, that isn't nice. There's no need to rub my issue in my face. I'm putting my hands up and saying I had a problem with alcohol. I'm sharing something personal and a failing on my part. It's embarrassing, and it's not something I wanted to have consume my life.

So, to have people shout from the rooftops in my face they don't have this issue themselves makes me feel a bit shitty about myself.

I appreciate it isn't their intention though and some are trying to justify their own actions and they're dealing with their own issues with alcohol.

As I started to tell people about my addiction to alcohol, I wondered whether I was making a big deal out of something small. I don't want to make light of something that is an incredibly difficult, and in many cases, tragic disease for so many mums and families globally.

The Australian Bureau of Statistics says:

"Alcohol-related fatalities extend beyond those deaths which are directly attributable to alcohol. In 2017 there were 4,186 deaths where alcohol was mentioned as being a contributing factor to mortality.

For deaths of females registered in 2017, a standardised rate of 7.0 deaths per 100,000 persons was recorded and represents the highest mortality rate of alcohol-related deaths for females in twenty years.

Deaths due to injury, (including suicide, transport accidents and falls), were the most common underlying causes of death to have alcohol mentioned as a contributory factor."

I'm glad I shared my story because it has opened my eyes to how significant this issue has been in my life and how damaging it was without me realising. Even in the early days of me quitting, I didn't realise what a transformation this would have on my life and my health, and particularly on my mental health. And again, so many other mums have come forward to me now and said they share the same issue they want to do something about it.

This is important. It's an important issue to talk about. It's important for me to talk about it because it's therapeutic in many ways. And it also helps me to connect with others who have either done the same thing, overcome the same challenge or are potentially thinking about it.

I'm still surprised at how many other mums have come forward since and told me they have been struggling too.

So many mums. And especially mums in the early years of their businesses who work for themselves from home as I do.

Or they'll tell me they've struggled in the past and they also quit drinking for the same reasons.

But they tell me they're struggling right now, and they don't know how to stop. They asked me for my advice on how I did it. Many picked up the Allen Carr book too and have stayed in touch to let me know how their journey is going. It was a big surprise to me, that I wasn't alone.

Eva, who I told you about previously, is a mother of two who also manages mental health matters. Her doctors had prescribed medication to help her, but alcohol was preventing the medication from doing its job.

She said:

"I'm over 100 days sober and it's changed my life. Alcohol, my mental illness and medication didn't mix, and it destroyed all hope of me feeling good. Now I know what good feels like on and even on a bad day, I don't think about alcohol. Alcohol doesn't rule my life anymore and I'm over the moon."

Alcohol was preventing Eva from feeling better, as it had been me when it stopped me from fighting my real demons.

Mum of two young children, Sara told me:

"Since you stopped drinking and have talked about it so much; it's made me reflect a lot on my drinking habits. I know towards the end of last year I was drinking more than I normally would and drinking most nights, not just 2-3 times a week."

Are mothers especially susceptible to increased alcohol consumption?

In my circle of friends, this could the case. But that said, most of my friends are now mothers.

My friend Niamh said:

"I probably have a gin and tonic maybe two or three times a week after the kids are in bed. Usually only one, but if I've had a stressful day, I feel like I "deserve" it and it unwinds me. Your decision to stop drinking, plus the current sober movement is definitely making me question myself and think about my motives though."

My susceptibility to become addicted to alcohol wasn't just a response to the PTSD and anxiety that came after my cancer diagnosis. I wonder if society pushes the belief mums *should* drink to relax.

I think about the high number of wine-drinking inspired memes on social media and I know I've also been guilty in the past of creating and sharing some of those too.

It's a common language between many mums, the glue that binds us together in the trenches of motherhood. Alcohol.

All the mummy wine memes about wine always being the answer to every mums' struggles.

Example: "Q = (blank space), A = Wine".

Oh, how I laughed at that one, telling my friends it would go viral on social media. And it did. The mums in my community understood it and it spoke to them, as it had to me.

Some of them could relate to wine being the answer and there didn't seem to be anything wrong with associating ourselves with that phrase because we all thought it. If we're all doing it and we're all saying it's ok, then it is, right?

But for some of us, or all of us, it isn't ok. And it wasn't for me anymore.

I googled "sober mum memes" to see what inspiration I could find for staying alcohol-free and you know what came up?

"Being a mom is fun, but I could never do it sober."

"The most expensive part of having kids (picture of woman drinking huge glass of wine) is all the wine you have to drink."

"Oops!!! Did I buy wine instead of milk again?"

These were the first few results, and I had to stop looking then.

Confessing to my family and friends I was overcoming my secret addiction to alcohol was therapeutic. But it also made me question if society accepts, and often pushes, the message alcohol dependency in mothers is ok.

I'll share with you the experiences of other mums who've quit alcohol later but next, let's revisit those fears I talked about pre-sobriety.

LIFE AFTER ALCOHOL

Do you remember at the start of the book I confided some fears I had about quitting the booze?

Would I be boring?

Would my confidence wane?

Would I still be able to be around people who were drinking?

Would I still enjoy... karaoke?

Well, let me tell you how I've faced those fears so far and it truly is liberating to know I'm now not tied to alcohol. I don't limit myself to only visiting restaurants that serve alcohol.

I can drive anywhere at any time because I'm never over the limit.

I know no matter how long I take to get to sleep, or how little I sleep, I won't have the added symptoms of a hangover the next day.

I know every day I'm thinking a little less about drinking and freeing up more space in my mind, my day and my life to do other things. Things more important for my life and mission. I'm free and I have much more time.

You know what though, I'm not just surviving life without wine, I'm thriving because of it.

I'll share with you how four main areas of my life improved when I stopped drinking alcohol. They were my:

- Family Life
- Career
- Finances
- Health

I'd expected that both my physical and mental health would improve, and it was the driving force behind what I stopped drinking.

But there have been so many other unexpected changes I hadn't bargained for.

Family Life

These days, I'm a more mindful mum.

When I go to bed now, I'm clear-headed and sober. That means if for any reason in the day or night I need to drive my kids to the hospital or out of danger, I can.

And yes, I know it's drastic, but it was one of the biggest contributors to the anxiety I felt every single night I drank.

The guilt if they needed me, I might not be there for them.

I'm also much more present in their lives now. I no longer hang out for '7pm wine time' which means if I'm with my kids, at work or doing something alone, I commit to that moment and I'm mindful of being there.

I hear more; I see more and I'm happier. The foggy headedness has gone, and I take in more of my children's little lives and commit those memories to my mind, confident they won't be so quickly forgotten.

I feel like a good mum again.

The hangover included anxiety I felt wasn't always rational. Sometimes, it led to me feeling like I wasn't enough for my kids when I was. I'm always here for them and they're growing into well-rounded, independent beautiful souls and I have a lot to do with that, as their mum.

I'm spending more time with them and congratulating myself and my husband on doing a great job.

Mindfulness and alcohol work both ways, it seems.

In a 2017 study published in the International Journal of Neuropsychopharmacology, University College London found practicing mindfulness for just eleven minutes per day helps heavy drinkers to cut back.

Dr Sunjeev Kamboj (UCL Clinical Psychopharmacology Unit), the study's lead author, said:

"We found that a very brief, simple exercise in mindfulness can help drinkers cut back, and the benefits can be seen quite quickly."

During the study, instead of suppressing their cravings, they paid attention to them and sat with them without acting on them.

Participants in the study who practiced mindfulness "drank 9.3 fewer units of alcohol (roughly equivalent to three pints of beer) in the following week compared to the week preceding the study."

Dr Kamboj said:

"Practising mindfulness can make a person more aware of their tendency to respond reflexively to urges. By being more aware of their cravings, we think the study participants were able to bring intention back into the equation, instead of automatically reaching for the drink when they feel a craving."

I'm (arguably) a better wife.

I'm more present for my husband too and we talk more in the evenings rather than drink together in silence.

Our lack of talking was leading to problems we need not have faced and I'm glad to be making some proactive steps in strengthening our relationship even more.

At times, these sober conversations lead to the odd heated debate but that's ok. Better to argue out our issues and resolve them than drink them away or hide them.

Career

The benefits I've experienced aren't all physical. One huge change I've seen is how much I've advanced at work.

I'm better at my job.

Since I now sleep better and my mind is clearer, my productivity and creativity has soared.

I haven't felt this motivated and inspired in years. While I'm never been short of ideas to grow my business; I now have the time and determination to stop procrastinating and get it done.

In fact, I hadn't realised how much the alcohol, well hangovers, had been affected my mood at work and how that led to my creativity being dulled.

I now wake up refreshed with a clear plan for each day and I'm ticking off my To-do list in triple time.

The goals I set at the start of the year are already

happening for me because I have so much less stress and so much more purpose.

I'm achieving more.

I don't just want to work; I want to excel. And I'm proud of everything I'm achieving now and more confident in shouting about it.

My ability to remember things was hugely affected after undergoing chemo and the resulting PTSD that stemmed from it. However, now I'm giving myself the best chance to remember because I have a clearer mind and really listen and take notice.

My mind is not drifting to the dark and tempting places it once was. I remember more and I forget less.

And because of this, I'm a more reliable colleague, partner and employee.

Finances

I've saved a small fortune.

The Australian Bureau of Statistics, in their Household Expenditure Survey reported that Australians spent $14.9b on alcohol purchases in 2016. That's compared to $1.6b on tea and coffee.

Source:https://www.abs.gov.au/AUSSTATS/abs@.nsf/Lookup/6530.0Main+Features12015-16?OpenDocument

The app I've been using, "I Am Sober" has a clever calculator to let me know how much money I've saved since quitting alcohol.

You enter the amount you were spending each week

and as time goes on; it adds it all up and my count is running well into the hundreds.

Seeing the amount I might have completely wasted on cheap wine keeps me motivated to continue.

Along with the healthier food choices, we're also spending way less on takeaways and the unhealthy snacks we would inhale during our boozy Netflix sessions.

In the past few months, we've already saved over $1000 on food and drink alone.

Since I'm now more focused, productive and creative at work, I'm also earning more.

I'm more confident in declining work that isn't in line with my goals and freeing up time and energy to focus on what will bring me closer to reaching them.

Health

1 sleep better.

I've mentioned a few times the positive impact quitting booze has had on my sleep and I'll rave some more.

Now, I sleep. Really sleep. Proper, deep, out-for-the-count sleep.

I'd struggled with insomnia since my teen years. After having kids, sleep deprivation was constant. When I finally fell asleep, the babies would wake me within minutes.

When they got older and slept for longer, I still struggled with staying asleep. I slept so lightly, and I swear if they rolled over or so much as sighed I woke up. I put it down to 'being a mum'.

Except now that's changed. I still sometimes struggle

with getting to sleep but once I'm out, I am OUT. I'm still an insomniac, but I'm sleeping better overall.

I'm reducing my risk of cancer.

I'll never know what caused my cancer and I suspect it was genetics. However, Cancer Council NSW says:

"Alcohol use is a cause of cancer. Any level of alcohol consumption increases the risk of developing an alcohol-related cancer; the level of risk increases in line with the level of consumption."

This is enough to solidify my decision to quit.

Cancer Council Australia says "There is strong evidence that alcohol use increases the risk of cancers of the mouth, pharynx, larynx, oesophagus, stomach, bowel, liver and breast.

Alcohol use may contribute to weight (fat) gain, and greater body fatness is a convincing cause of cancers of the oesophagus, pancreas, gallbladder, stomach, bowel, endometrium, ovary, kidney, liver, breast (in post-menopausal women) and prostate (advanced).

Source:https://www.cancercouncil.com.au/2397/about-us/our-annual-reports-and-research-activity-reports/our-position-statements-about-cancer-council-nsw/alcohol-and-cancer2/?pp=61362&cc=9160&&ct=35

I cannot rewrite the past, but I can protect my future health and I feel quitting alcohol is one thing I can do to minimise the risk of my cancer returning. Time will tell, but psychologically, it brings back some of the control whipped away from me when I was diagnosed.

I'm less anxious.

That 'next-day guilt' or paranoia or disappointment in myself has gone. Gone.

No more 'What did I do last night?' Or 'Why did I not stop drinking earlier?' Or 'Why did I do it again?'

I now wake up feeling fresh (ish), guilt-free and focused.

And I don't make stupid decisions or let myself fall into the wrong situations. I know what I'm doing now, all the time.

Beyond Blue says, "Some people use drugs or alcohol because they think they will make them feel better, but they can leave you feeling worse – anxious and agitated, or flat, unmotivated and moody. Your sense of reality can be affected too."

Source: https://www.beyondblue.org.au/the-facts/drugs-alcohol-and-mental-health

Anxiety and PTSD after cancer is still a *thing* for me. Still something I'm working on every day. But the anxiety I was giving myself from drinking too much, too frequently, has gone. And it feels amazing to be taking back some control in my life when so much has been taken away from me.

I make healthier food choices.

I didn't quit drinking to lose weight, but I expected the weight to fall off when I stopped. It hasn't and in fact, I've put on a few kilos.

This has really surprised me because the calories I was consuming through alcohol would have been massive.

However, I've changed my diet considerably, and it's

still early days. And despite putting on a bit of weight, the benefits of being sober from alcohol far outweigh the cons (pun totally intended!) so far.

I also *feel* healthier physically and being more clear-headed means I'm making better food choices.

So, whilst we still indulge in the odd takeaway (or vegan Magnum), it's less frequent and I've rekindled my love for cooking.

I look better.

When I look back on photographs and videos of myself before I became sober, I can see a real difference.

I've had numerous comments from friends about how my skin glows more now and I know that's a combination of subtracting alcohol, adding plants and getting more sleep.

My friend Niamh told me:

"You look bloody amazing so that just goes to show it was a good decision if you can see it so easily in your skin, eyes and general 'brightness'."

Unfortunately, my dark circles are hereditary but overall, and very quickly, I started to look brighter.

I feel better.

I no longer have hangovers and it still surprises me to realise I never will again. I think back to the hangovers of my past and think 'why?'

What about that wine was worth doing that to my body and my mind? And doing mum life with hangovers is a crappy combo.

And I know the answer is nothing. I can see now no event or memory in my life was made better by drinking my way through it. Absolutely none.

I would have still laughed, danced, hugged, talked, enjoyed and sang just as much but without the resulting hangover, paranoia, guilt and anxiety that inevitably came each time.

I no longer feel thirsty—physically or metaphorically. I'm hydrated and fulfilled.

I'm not keeping any more secrets. My biggest one is out. And despite the revelation that so many others shared in it, that hasn't normalised it for me.

I was lying to myself and others when I thought I didn't have a problem. I'm honest now. It feels good.

And I'm not alone.

In a 2019 study, the University of Melbourne asked new mothers about their drinking habits.

"Most women dramatically reduce their alcohol intake on learning they are pregnant, but by the time their child is five they are back to their pre-pregnancy drinking levels."

The paper, 'Alcohol and parenthood: an integrative analysis of the effects of transition to parenthood in three Australasian cohorts' is published in the latest edition of *Drug and Alcohol Dependence* journal.

This is in line with my life. I didn't drink any alcohol during my pregnancies, and only a tiny amount during the six months I breastfed each baby.

However, over the years, I've ramped up my drinking so much I was drinking even more than before I had kids.

So, despite staying in the kids and the vast reduction in

social events since becoming a mother, my drinking levels didn't dip over time.

I'm interested in the connection between motherhood and alcohol generally, not just for new mothers.

It led me to conduct my own survey and I'll share the results with you next.

MOTHERHOOD AND ALCOHOL – WHY DO MUMS DRINK?

Becoming more aware of my own issues with alcohol opened my eyes to the subject overall. I'm not alone with this. I'm not the first mother in the world to turn to alcohol too many times for the wrong reasons and fall butt-first into the alcohol trap with no clear path to crawl back out.

In my circle of friends alone, I see and hear from so many of them who are struggling with the same issue.

I see some are drinking to relax but they're sometimes in a frantic state to get there as quickly as possible. They're panicking they'll be the 'soberest'. They want to blend in ASAP and the last train known as alcohol is about to leave the station.

And I was doing this, constantly on my feet getting the next round in or heading to the bar or the kitchen for a refill.

Drinking frantically to relax.

Of course, not all the mums I know have an addiction to alcohol! Some are perfectly happy with their consumption and some want to cut back a little. Or to be more mindful about the reasons they're drinking.

Although, when I started sharing my story on my blog and social media, it overwhelmed me how many other mothers reached out to say, "Me too, Mim".

It's what led me to want to learn more and to uncover more insights into the link between motherhood and alcohol and the reasons behind why other mums drink.

The Motherhood & Alcohol 2019 Survey

I had my own notions about why mothers drink alcohol or not and I based these views purely on my own beliefs, experiences and those in my circle of mum friends.

It wasn't enough, and I wanted to know more, so I decided a survey would get me the answers I was looking for.

This isn't a science experiment or a university study, people, so let's kick aside the soapboxes before you leap on. That said, it's insightful and a great guide. It fascinated me.

In my anonymous survey of 1000 mothers, I asked them these main questions around their drinking habits:

1. Do you drink alcohol?
2. What alcoholic drinks do you consume most frequently?
3. Why do you consume alcoholic drinks?
4. How often do you drink alcohol?
5. Where do you consume alcohol most frequently?
6. How many standard drinks (units) of alcohol do you drink each week?
7. Has the amount you drink changed since becoming a mother?
8. Do you think the media/social media perpetuates the message that mothers drink a lot of alcohol?
9. Approximately, how much do you spend on alcohol

purchases each week?
10. Are you happy with the amount of alcohol you currently drink?

I first asked them some demographic questions to build up a picture about their family such as how many children they have, their kids' ages and their age.

Survey Results

Let's explore the results, starting with the demographics:

Are you a mother?

1000 said yes. 1 said no. I removed the latter from the rest of the results therefore these results are based upon 1000 mothers' responses.

Where do you live?

Response	%
Australia	83.80
New Zealand	1.80
United Kingdom	9.20
United States	3.10
Canada	0.90
Other	1.20

How old are you?

Response	%
Under 19	0
20-29	9.20
30-39	48.20
40-49	36.30
50-59	5.50
60+	0.80

How many children do you have?

Response	%
1	21.80
2	49.80
3	20.30
4	5.80
5+	2.30

How old are your children?

Response	%
Currently Pregnant	3.50
0-2	36.90
3-5	42.50
6-10	45.60
11-15	27.80
16+	15.60

What's your total household income? (In Australian Dollars)

Response	%
Under $50,000	12.00
$50,000 to $99,999	28.00
$100,000 to $149,999	30.60
$150,000 to 199,999	15.10
$200,000+	14.30

What is your work status?

Response	%
I am not employed	20.30
I work for someone else	53.20
I work for myself (own business)	18.00
I work for myself and for someone else	8.50

We'll now move on to the questions relating to alcohol consumption. For many of the questions, I asked for expansion. I wanted to know more details on why they answered as they did, and I'll share these further insights in the next chapters.

Do you drink alcohol?

Response	%
Yes	82.50
No	17.50

For the mothers who replied No, I asked them to provide further details on why they choose not to drink alcohol.

What alcoholic drinks do you consume most frequently?

Response	%
Wine	64.60
Gin	15.10
Vodka	10.20
Cider	15.80
Beer	16.20
Cocktails	9.10
Pre-mixed drinks	9.60
I do NOT drink alcoholic drinks	14.30
Other (respondents specified)	7.10

I provided the most common options I knew of and asked them to add their own. Whiskey, bourbon, rum and Champagne were the most common additions.

Why do you consume alcoholic drinks?

Response	%
To relax	63.80
It's a habit	16.60
I like the taste	53.20
To get drunk	7.00
It's expected socially	13.30
I am persuaded by adverts for alcohol	0.30
To gain confidence	5.10
I do NOT drink alcoholic drinks	14.40

This was the question I was most interested in looking at the data on and 293 mothers responded with further insights.

How often do you drink alcohol?

Response	%
Every day	8.00
A few times a week	25.10
Weekends only	13.30
A few times a month	15.20
Once a month	6.70
Less than once a month	18.50
I do NOT drink alcoholic drinks	13.20

Where do you consume alcohol most frequently?

Response	%
Home	63.30
Bar	4.30
Friend's House	5.30
Work	0.50
Event (e.g. wedding, party, birthday)	11.00
I do NOT drink alcoholic drinks	13.30
Other	2.30

Most people who provided clarification for Other said it was in a Restaurant.

How many standard drinks (units) of alcohol do you drink each week?

Response	%
0-3	47.70
4.7	19.00
8-14	11.30
15+	5.80
I do NOT drink alcoholic drinks	16.20

Has the amount you drink changed since becoming a mother?

Response	%
I now drink more	19.50
I now drink less	52.00
I drink the same amount	17.90
I do NOT drink alcoholic drinks	10.60

I requested further clarification from this question and captured 307 further insights from the mothers who used to drink before becoming a mother and have since stopped, or vice versa.

Do you think that the media/social media perpetuates the message that mothers drink a lot of alcohol? (e.g. TV or magazine ads, Facebook memes etc)

Response	%
Yes	61.00
No	25.70
Don't know	13.30

289 mothers provided further commentary around this.

Approximately how much do you spend on alcoholic purchases each week? (in Australian Dollars)

Response	%
$0-14	47.90
$15-29	18.70
$30-44	9.80
$45-59	4.90
$60+	4.10
I do NOT drink alcoholic drinks	14.60

Are you happy with the amount of alcohol you currently drink?

Response	%
Yes	62.40
No – I would rather drink less	23.70
No – I would rather drink more	2.30
I do NOT drink alcoholic drinks	11.60

206 mothers responded further commentary.

Finally, I asked respondents if they had more to add to the conversation. I wanted their comments and opinions on the alcohol consumption of mothers and their own experiences relating to this.

226 respondents provided more info.

Now, I could use these comments to skew my book. I could back up my decision to quit alcohol, and the reasons behind it, with literally hundreds of comments.

But I'll provide balance where it exists.

In the next chapter, I'll lay out some experiences and opinions other mothers have. Why they do, or don't drink. It's eye-opening.

Further Insights from the Survey

The most helpful part of examining the survey results for me was uncovering the stories behind the answers.

Whilst some survey responses are 'black and white' and can be taken at face value, so many needed more. More knowledge, more substance.

As the survey was anonymous, I'm comfortable sharing some of these insights with you now.

Question 8 - Do you drink alcohol?

Let's dive deeper. I asked those respondents who answered No to this question to provide further info, and many stated they didn't like the taste, the hangovers, were pregnant/breastfeeding or had never drank much alcohol.

Here is a collection of some other notable responses:

"I was addicted to it."

"After both of my sons died, I felt out-of-control and lost. Alcohol made it worse, so I stopped drinking."

"Never have. Don't like the idea of being dependent on something to get through."

"I'm currently pregnant but I haven't been a big drinker anyway. My mum was an alcoholic and I think it has affected the way I see and look at alcohol. I don't like effects."

"Need to be in control to supervise my children."

"Alcohol became a very destructive part of my lifestyle before I fell pregnant (the reason I fell pregnant) and I decided from the moment I found out I was pregnant that I would not drink alcohol again."

"I simply never started as a teenager because I hated seeing all my friends getting drunk."

"Have had cancer and have lynch syndrome so do not want to increase by chances of getting it again."

"Don't agree with drinking whilst caring for young children. My youngest is in remission from leukaemia and at any point we might need to go to A&E. It would put his life at risk to drink and be incapacitated or unable to drive. But I was against drink before his diagnosis for the same reason, in case of an emergency I think it's just irresponsible."

"I feel awful when I drink it. I don't have time for a hangover. I want to be present for the kids. My parents are alcoholics."

"I have a few... I don't really enjoy it; I feel drowsy and who needs that? Alcoholism runs in the family and I don't want my son to think drinking is no big deal. For him, it could be a very big deal. IF I'm able to keep him from trying alcohol until after he's twenty-one, his chances of developing the disease will be dramatically less. :)"

"As I got older, alcohol started to make me very aggressive and a mean and nasty drunk. Once I had kids, I decided that I didn't want to get up to a crying baby with a hangover."

"Our culture has an unhealthy attachment and

perceived need to have alcohol."

"I don't like the taste much, and I know that I tend to just binge drink on a night out on very rare occasions. I don't like drinking alone, it's a social thing. I hate that it makes me feel so tired."

"It makes me want to sleep; I like to drive everywhere so I don't risk drinking."

"It does not interest me at all since having children."

"It's like a drug."

"Religious reasons."

"I never drank much anyway (there are plenty of non-alcoholic drinks I preferred, and which were cheaper), so it was easy to stop when we started trying to get pregnant. Then just haven't started again."

"I just don't anymore. It's not good for you, it's a waste of money and I was sick of every social event revolving around alcohol as much if my family is heavy drinkers."

"I grew up in a family who never had alcohol because my mother's uncles were all alcoholics and she did not like what happened to them. Coincidentally my husband also grew up in a family that didn't drink at all, so we just never started. These days it concerns me how much drinking is used as a crutch in our culture and I don't waste to be a part of that."

"I'd rather be in complete control when responsible for my children. I've never been a big drinker anyway."

"Don't like the taste of it and can't stand people being idiots when drinking."

"I was married to an alcoholic for twenty years and the impact of his drinking on every aspect of our lives was horrific. I have chosen not to drink alcohol because I feel it has no positive effect on my life."

Question 10 - Why do you consume alcoholic drinks?

Besides the options I had given, I asked them to add further commentary. The results here were fascinating, many echoing the reasons I used to drink. There were further reasons given that I found unexpected:

"A drink at the end of the day can give me the energy needed to make it through the battle for bedtime."

"Particularly after a stressful day, which usually has more to do with the children than my business... sadly."

"I feel like I drink more out of habit than anything - it's almost automatic to pour a glass of wine whilst cooking dinner - I don't usually even think about whether or not I "feel" like a wine. When I go out socially, I drink to ease social anxiety- I am very shy and have trouble talking to people, a glass of wine (or 2) always seems to help."

"I used to drink to self-medicate when I lived in another country. Now I enjoy a drink at the end of the day, not as excessively but there are days when it feels like the glass is a coping mechanism for how I feel internally about being a mum and not feeling okay about things."

"I am an adult. I am in control of the decisions I make for myself. If I like something, I will enjoy it."

"After my little girl is in bed and all the chores have been done, I will sometimes sit down with a glass of wine and watch some TV."

"I'm a single mother. Once the children are both asleep, I generally get an hour or so to relax before I'm falling asleep."

"After a long day it is nice to relax with a glass of red

wine... albeit I think it is habitual."

"I'm breastfeeding, so I will occasionally have half a glass of red. That's about it. My drinking habits have certainly changed since becoming a mother!"

"Kids teatime is my favourite time for a glass of wine. It helps me to relax and I feel I deserve it! After kids' bedtime I might have one more or just a cup of tea. I'm over it by then. But a 6pm glass helps me through!! I try to have at least 2 days a week with no alcohol."

"To escape."

"Saturday night, wine night! I love a couple of drinks to unwind. When I meet friends to catch up, we have a drink, it's just how it is. This is wrong really, but it's just how it is."

"I tend to drink (one drink only) on extra stressful days - it helps me relax, manage my anxiety, and ensure that I respond calmly to any further stressors. On the days my husband is home, I will often have one drink with him to wind down in the evening - basically, I drink because he drinks. I don't drink every day, but I do find myself looking forward to the taste and relaxation. I will decline a drink on many days when I know having water or tea will better serve my health and wellbeing."

"I'm really only a social drinker (to excess) or if I've been through something stressful. Also, a red wine sometimes on the weekend when the fire is on."

"It's definitely talked a lot about in my mother's group which does encourage me to have a drink."

"It is something to look forward to at the end of a long day of housework, food prep, drop offs and a full-time job it is something to look forward to. It breaks the monotony of being at home every night as well."

"I have recently become single and only see my children during the week. Because I am lonely and want to be around people, I will go out to the bar and talk with whoever is there."

"I drank to numb my feels. Some days it would be one drink, some days none other days too many and I shouldn't have been in charge of children. It was never that I was falling over drunk every day it was more recognising the reasons I drank and when I drank. I drank more than I needed, and it was never in company especially since having children. Historically, pre-kids and marriage I was a binge drinker and I would drink to black out. I was raped a number of times when I was too drunk to consent or otherwise, and there were times that I was drunk and got myself into unwilling sexual situations. Alcohol could have ruined my life. There was also a period of drugs and an addiction to money. All these things are to numb the feelings of life to push it all down so that I simply don't have to think or feel. It doesn't work and it solves none of those issues but still I did it."

"One glass of red wine seems to slow things down around me. It makes me feel warm and I don't feel as highly strung. If I go out and there is alcohol served, then my motivation is more to be social, gain confidence in a group, to let go and be silly."

"Being a young mum and the first of my friends to have a baby, my friends are still young and often have parties where it is expected to drink. It's nice to feel normal and a part of the group still. I just don't overdo it because I know I have my son to look after and he comes first."

"I find I'm a better person to be around and less highly strung if I have a drink or 2 around 4pm to kick off the evening chaos of homework, meal prep, nagging, baths, dishes and the fighting that comes with having 3 boys!"

"I'm a mum of 4, 3 who live with me, all with special needs of some form. I have the occasional glass of wine to relax. Sometimes I drink a whole bottle in a night!"

"I feel that it is implied that you cannot have fun unless you drink. Also, I worry about how many parents use alcohol as a coping mechanism to deal with kids and how it seems socially acceptable to do it."

"I enjoy having a few drinks to relax and chill with hubby. We have awesome chats when we are both having a few drinks together. It brings us closer as a couple and let's be honest the sex is better. 😊 I haven't had many drinking nights since May 2016 due to being pregnant and breastfeeding 2 babies."

"I've had a long history of using alcohol as a tool to de-stress. This is SO unhealthy and something that I am still battling with. Whilst I am no longer as bad as I was before I was a mother, when I drink with the sole purpose of 'getting drunk' things have ended pretty messily. I only really have that motivation when I have been feeling highly stressed for a period of time. Mostly, I only have a drink or two, maybe once a fortnight, sometimes on a Friday after work, and usually after I play a game of soccer on a Saturday. But when I binge drink with the purpose of getting drunk, it tends to be a lot more than that in the space of a few hours. This usually coincides with me wanting to go to the pub which spirals in to drinking for confidence and/or to alleviate mum guilt!"

"I find myself wanting a drink when the stress of kids whinging, and cooking dinner gets too much. I'm also dealing with marriage problems and have been drinking more than usual."

"These days, I drink because I enjoy it and I generally only drink wine. I enjoy the taste and I won't drink bad wine – call me a snob! I like a glass of wine whilst I'm cooking dinner, mainly at the weekends but occasionally during the week and the most I'll have is two glasses at a time."

Question 14 - Has the amount you drink changed since becoming a mother?

307 mothers wanted to say more about their response to this question and why their drinking habits have changed since they became a mum:

"Far less. I realised being pregnant that I can be social without drinking, trying to parent hungover is the worst, I also just think if one of my kids got sick overnight and needed to go to the hospital imagine having to call an ambulance/someone else to get them because you're too drunk to drive. 😬"

"I used to drink every day but have cut down a lot as I just wasn't able to function. I was grumpy, short and intolerable. Now I'm nice and calm. I'm hoping to quit altogether."

"When my child was diagnosed with a chronic disease, I drank more then as a coping mechanism. Have since cut back as I feel better and sleep better with less alcohol."

"I drink less, but more often."

"It's more about age than motherhood."

"My friends drink and seems more and more acceptable to drink and joke about 'wine o'clock' is 5pm."

"Having young children is difficult. I drink more now

they are in school, and it is at the end of the day, whilst cooking dinner and getting the children sorted."

"Before I was a mum, I used to go out most weekends and would drink until the early hours of the morning. Now I have a couple of drinks at home before going to bed at 9pm. 😄"

"I was a binge drinker before having my children and would frequently go out at the weekend. I can't survive my children with a hangover and as the only adult in the house I obviously can't get drunk."

"I don't like to be drunk around my children, I had alcoholic parents and I don't want to be that for my kids."

"Now my children are older I'm able to socialise with friends on a regular basis again. Inevitably we set the world to rights over a bottle of wine!"

"Since having our son, my husband and I now get a takeout and a bottle of wine on a Friday as a way to relax at the end of a busy week."

"I have always been conscious of how alcohol affects me both mentally and physically, so I still use the same criteria to decide whether to drink - do I really need help relaxing/being more comfortable in a social situation? Or would my body feel better if I hydrated with water/chamomile tea? Since becoming a mom, I'm in far fewer social situations so I drink less in one sitting, but my overall stress has increased. So there are more days of the week when I'll have a drink to mellow out, so I think it averages out to drinking the same amount each week!"

"Since becoming a mum, I drink more midweek than weekends."

"I drink far less now than I did before. I don't have the same social occasions to go out and drink with friends. I'm more health conscious now I'm a mum, and I've got young eyes watching me."

"I used to go out and get drunk before kids. When my kids were first born, I didn't drink at all. Over the years I've found I enjoy a wine or two at night. Mostly Friday's but also a couple of nights a week I'll have a glass. If I'm dieting though, wine is the first to go. I guess you could say my alcohol usage is up and down depending on what I'm doing in life."

"I drink most days but never get drunk or use alcohol to have a good time. It is now more a relaxant, a habit and something to look forward to at the end of a long day, none of which contains any time for myself. A couple of glasses at the end of the day is my reward."

"I hate feeling like crap when I'm with my child and the less I drink the less tolerance I have."

"Since my late twenties the amount I drink has become less and less as I get older and even more since becoming a mother."

"During my pregnancy I stopped drinking for obvious reasons and just haven't seemed to feel the urge or need to drink again."

"I didn't start to drink wine because children are stressful, it had more to do with my maturity and wanting to try different things and appreciating the taste of wine. I didn't really like the taste in my twenties."

"I don't want my children thinking that the only way to have fun is by drinking. I'm very mindful to show them."

"I don't have time to drink alcohol. I work at a paid job, get homework (washing, tidying, taxiing, cooking, cleaning up dinner, getting kids to bed) sleeping then going to work. 😕"

"I drink every night (at least a couple of glasses). Before kids it was just on the weekend."

"I'm more aware of health impacts of drinking since having kids, and of the impact of them seeing me drinking, so since becoming a mum I've reduced the amount I drink. My partner drinks a lot so I also want my kids to see that alcohol doesn't have to be a part of everyday."

"Because my son doesn't understand the concept of sleep ins!!"

"I think I also have more disposable income now too, and therefore more to spend on luxuries like alcohol. (Or I could be trying to rationalise my habits...)"

"I don't 'binge' drink any more like I did when I was younger."

"Not working full time made additional days feel like 'weekends'."

"Since I spend so many evenings in, I do drink a bit more than before having babies. It feels a bit like a treat and a way to reward myself when I've had a tiring day. Before kids I might have been more inclined to go out, work out, or do an activity that was not necessarily linked to alcohol."

"Early evening is my worst time.... dealing with post school kids and evening routine."

"I'm way more stressed and use alcohol to unwind. Especially with another mother friend."

"I used to drink much more before I was a mum. Friday - Sunday but never weeknights! Now I have a few on weeknights and weekends but don't get plastered like I used to!"

"Not appropriate to be under the influence when

responsible for children."

Question 15 - Do you think that the media/social media perpetuates the message that mothers drink a lot of alcohol?

Ok, I was looking forward to reading through the 289 comments that came with this one. Would my opinion be supported or quashed?

And I'll admit the question holds some provocation. The responses though, had the majority saying Yes:

"There seems to be a view that mums need wine at the end of the day and that Gin will reward people after a busy day."

"In every TV show centred on mums, it's all about having a drink to relax."

"I think the wine/gin mum culture on social media is probably great solidarity for the few mums that enjoy a glass of wine after a rough day with kids. (Probably the healthiest easily accessible self-medication in our society; to a group of people- mothers - who are largely isolated/socially undervalued) but I don't think any benefit outweighs the unquestionable enabling it does for alcoholic mums. (Both those in the brink of alcoholism, those deep in it and those desperately trying to recover.)"

"It is everywhere! And touted as the only solution to every parenting woe."

"After reducing the amount I drink and trying to quit, I suddenly realised how much drinking was commented on, from the radio (whilst driving kids to school), social media, tv shows (Bad Mothers - Australia Netflix - they show them drinking constantly). It's advertised like a club that if you don't drink, you aren't a part of it. Even future women (who I got this survey from) have their drinks and social events. If I don't drink you feel like you are on the outer like being unpopular at school."

"There are plenty of articles discussing the drinking habits of mothers which I think are quick to shame."

"I don't see things like this on my social media, perhaps it's my own social group it's just not very present."

"I love the FB memes, and I am not on the bandwagon of how it glorifies drinking, it is light-hearted fun about the reality of a lot of women. We celebrate getting through another day with a glass of wine. For most people it is controlled, they can stop, and it is okay. I feel a minority may have an issue. Does it influence my drinking? No, not at all."

"I don't think social media claims mothers drink excessively but there does seem to be a perception that mothers NEED alcohol to relax and enjoy each other's company during an evening. I've been looked at in many a weird way for asking for a brew at a mums gathering when we're out... I'm 'out-out' to have an adult conversation and connect with people and I don't feel I HAVE to consume alcohol to do this. But if I feel like I'd enjoy that connection more if I had a drink I will."

"It's irresponsible to get drunk whilst the mum is looking after their child. Regardless of whether they're in bed. Just the one glass is OK. But there should be more awareness of alcoholism as dependency as a habit, even a small amount but regularly. This is damaging to both their physical and mental health."

"I think the media makes it out like a mum is a bad person for having a glass of wine."

"You see a lot of shops with glasses etc with the words 'mummy's juice', 'mummy's wine glass' etc."

"Wine mummy culture is everywhere, and it has recently started to concern me for personal health but mainly the message that send to kids."

"It is made out that the only way we can deal with motherhood stresses is to hit the bottle."

"Loads of Facebook memes, greetings cards, bloggers all seem to celebrate the fact that mums need to drink wine / gin / Prosecco, etc."

"I think the 'coffee to cocktails' trend has been normalised and encouraged as a viable method of self-care for mothers. It feels like you're almost expected to partake in that trend - like mothers have so much stress that they're not capable of surviving without coffee and cocktails. I wish that there was more support and encouragement for moms to partake in true self-care methods like helping moms not feel guilty about taking a little time to themselves or going out with friends or having a date night with their husband/partner."

"I think some mums also play up to this expectation. Although I do know of others that are basically alcoholics also."

"I don't buy into the social media BS."

"Mums often make it into a joke like they need wine to cope but it's not really very funny and sends a bad message to new mothers who might genuinely struggle but alcohol will make genuine struggles worse."

"I think it's self-perpetuated by mothers and mothers' groups. Alcohol advertising is prohibited, and I don't think mothers drinking would pass advertising standards. Perhaps in movies yes. But Facebook videos and memes I suspect are made by the target audience to foster a sense of camaraderie."

"I think social media and memes make me feel more comfortable about drinking. They make me think it's acceptable which I don't necessarily think is a good thing."

"I feel mothers make so many jokes about wine. There's nothing funny about needing alcohol to cope with the stresses that being a mother brings. I find it sad and disgusting."

"In mothers' groups on social media it seems the answer to everything is to have a glass of wine."

"I do, but I also think a lot of mums DO drink too much, so I guess there's no smoke without fire."

"It pisses me off, alcoholism isn't cute or funny, it's a problem."

"I don't really hear negative media on mums drinking."

"I'm always seeing things like mums need wine at the end of the day or to deal with their children. Xmas gift ideas for educators are always wine with funny labels such as sorry my kid is the reason you drink."

"The media are always displaying mothers drinking wine."

"It seems that mummy drinks more to cope with the stress of being a parent."

"I feel with all the memes that mothers are expected to drink. Especially in Australian culture. People assume I'm boring because I don't drink or that there's something wrong with me."

"Some bloggers on Facebook do kind of make out that motherhood and drinking go hand in hand."

"Social media mostly - lots of joke posts and memes

about mums drinking wine and gin."

"I think we are targeted to feel guilty. We are portrayed as "stressed so we drink", "glamorous so we drink" "dishevelled so we drink" "slovenly so we drink". Rarely are we portrayed as the masters of the entire family who actually are too intelligent to not be sensible about our alcohol choices & consumption."

"Never thought about it. I think a lot of comments I see from mums I know suggest they drink a lot."

"The stereotype of wine or gin every evening to unwind or making the most of kid free evenings out to let loose and get drunk."

"I think social media and companies assume all mums drink an insane amount of wine, which isn't true. It takes me a good week to go through a bottle of wine, and it usually goes flat before I can finish it, so I chuck it. Moms drink, but they don't normally drink ALL the time."

"The whole Mummy Wine Time culture is abhorrent. It is not normal for mothers or anyone to need a drink in order to function, let alone to be around their own children. It's disturbing to me and I don't participate in any memes or conversation that accepts that wine is necessary for me to be a calm and composed mother."

"It seems so normalised now. We have this faux self-care message going around that all of mummy's problems will be alleviated by a wine. I think at best, that disguises systemic issues around support for parents or the lack thereof."

"Too many high-profile mothers have made it seem ok."

"Mums supposedly survive on coffee during the day and wine once kids are in bed."

"I do in a way because some mothers make a lot of jokes about it but in my experience, the mothers I know that do make these jokes understand their limits and are not led by peers and social media. Having an alcoholic drink shouldn't be shamed and those who feel they need/crave/can't go without genuinely may need to think about the root cause. But I would have a hard time believing that mothers drink because they're mothers was accurate in every case."

"Stop it with the 'send wine' mum memes!"

"There is so much messaging that assumes that mothers drink A LOT of alcohol or that for some reason we MUST drink to survive being a parent... I don't drink to survive my kids..."

Question 17 - Are you happy with the amount of alcohol you currently drink?

206 mothers provided more insights to this and here are some responses:

"I would like to have less nights where I consume alcohol."

"I only drink on weekends and at social events... I've learned since becoming a mum that two drinks are ideal... three is a max... and anything more than that means dealing with the early rise/parental duties in the morning becomes all too hard!"

"Now that my children are getting older (5 & 7) and both at school, I feel like I have a more solid routine and are somewhat in more control with the day to day. I feel less reliant on alcohol to get me through the week. But there are still plenty of challenges!"

"I am reducing my alcohol intake. It is more for my health. I am clearer in the head, less irritable, able to cope better and feel good when I am alcohol-free. No doubt about that. But I enjoy a glass at night, and that is a marked improvement."

"I drink when I feel I want to, presently that's very rarely. I do wish sometimes that when I do drink it didn't affect me as much as it does. I used to be able to drink much more and not feel affected. Now it affects me quite quickly, so I tend to drink much less as I hate feeling drunk."

"I have cut down massively."

"It has contributed to extra weight gain after having 2 kids in 2 years."

"I don't want it to become a habit, and I don't want to teach my kids that is ok to drink every night."

"I love alcohol, but I make a real effort to drink no more than 14-18 units a week and to have 2 days off for my liver to recover."

"This is a hard one for me to answer. I'm torn between being ok with how much I drink because I really only go through one bottle of wine a week, and I enjoy each glass to the fullest. At the same time, I don't like that I do depend on a chemical to help me relax or get through a stressful day. However, I know that I am aware of my anxiety and triggers. I know that I'm always working to improve, and I do choose not to drink when I know I will feel better as a result. So I think for where I'm at right now, I am ok with how much I drink."

"I tend to drink a bit at parties or social occasions but I'm a bit of a hermit these days (anxiety) so it doesn't happen too often."

"I'd rather limit my alcohol usage to once a week. It's easy to get into the habit of a wine at night."

"I drink by the bottle at home... once a bottle is opened, I drink every night until it's gone... not an ideal situation."

"I'd love to give up. I'll definitely do dry July this year."

"I am not a heavy drinker, so am comfortable with my level. Red wine is good for you."

"Would like to cut back to minimise health risks, increase vitality and save money."

"My weight would probably be less if I drank less beer."

"I would happily never drink again."

"I feel that I have an unhealthy dependence on alcohol that scares me. I have noticed that when I'm in a group, I finish my glass of wine much quicker than everyone else."

"I would drink more if I had money to purchase."

"On certain occasions it would be nice to have more, but we still have children to look after, so I need to be able to be a responsible adult. If I couldn't drink at all then that wouldn't bother me either. I use it as a little treat at the end of the week to relax with my partner. It's kind of like dessert at the end of a meal, it's great to have but it's not always necessary."

"It sounds shameful that I drink so much. I know it's not doing me any favours, but at that time of the arvo, I find it really does help me get through the final leap of the day!"

"If we had a larger wine budget, I would probably be more consistent about wine with a daily meal, instead of wine with a meal once a week or so. I wouldn't mind more expensive wines either but since I can't always tell the difference, I've never really cared much."

"I like not drinking, but I do miss the feeling sometimes. Not of being drunk, but the warm, sleepy, tingly feeling you get BEFORE getting drunk."

"After many years of working on my relationship with alcohol, I feel that I am at a good place in my life with it and have been for some years now. I do not feel the need to drink every day, or any time I go out. As a matter of fact, if I am at a venue where there is no decent wine available, I am happy to drink a soft drink, coffee, etc. I really enjoy the voyage of discovery that food and wine can take a person on. I have even been able to share this with my son, which I feel will only serve to demystify alcohol for him and hopefully encourage his own healthy relationship with it into the future."

"I haven't had an alcoholic drink for 490 days. I gave up as I was drinking excessively for the sake of my mental and physical health."

"I've read all the research that says, basically, that no amount of alcohol is good for you. I take that on and wish I could go to zero. I have worked to reduce, but I do feel like there are few 'treats' and ways to enjoy a night in... so I'm working on it!"

"When I had my first child I drank heavily (1 or more bottles of wine at least 5 times a week) due to postnatal depression (diagnosed late). Until recently, I drank a little but since being diagnosed as bipolar and put on very strong meds, I can no longer drink."

Question 18 - Final Comments

And finally, I asked if any respondents had any further opinions or comments they would like to add to the conversation. I wanted to be sure to provide them with the opportunity to provide any balance or cover any areas of the subject the previous questions may not have, for them.

Out of the 226 responses, many expressed thanks in me raising the topic and looked forward to the results. Here are some notable responses:

"Motherhood is exhausting and I understand why some people choose to drink after a day of work/being at home with the kids. Personally, the hangover is not worth it for me. I'd rather go to the gym or knit than drink. There is definitely pressure to drink on nights out, but I am less susceptible to peer pressure than I once was, so I am happy to say no to a drink now, and not FOMO (fear of missing out)."

"I am more conscious of my drinking as my daughter hates the smell. I remember that smell from my own childhood when we would visit my parents' friends. Also, because I don't want her to form the opinion that alcohol is an emotional crutch and required to deal with stress."

"It's such a shame that marketers are using the "be in a group", "be Liked", "it's ok" to sell their product. Alcohol is just rammed down our throats and it's on the top of the list as far as worse drugs to take, yet it is sold as socially unacceptable to not drink. Women aren't told about the amount of cancers from alcohol and other sicknesses, or that it's a depressant. The government just keeps making money of alcohol and cigarettes yet bans other drugs (marijuana) that they cannot tax."

"I definitely feel like I am more responsible with my own alcohol consumption now I'm a mum purely with knowing I have to wake up with my parent hat on and can't afford a hangover. My husband owns a pub and so we are surrounded by alcohol all the time, but I've even noticed he's really cut back on drinking during the week as well. I do feel though that there is a narrative of mums who crack open a bottle every night to drink as a coping mechanism."

"Don't like to judge other mothers for how much they drink."

"My view is it would be irresponsible to be drunk looking after children. Mine used to wake often during the night and I wanted to attend to them. Alcohol can make me sleepy. One of my children had a couple of febrile convulsions when a very young child and I would check on home and my other children regularly. Alcohol may impair my functioning to do this."

"I think mothers need to drink less and teach their children to not drink too much. Also, it's awkward, uncomfortable and embarrassing, and possibly dangerous for the children when their parents are drunk."

"Wine culture needs to change. I need to reduce how much I drink to be healthier for myself and a better role model."

"My mum had a drinking problem for a few years and my father was an alcoholic. For me, being present and conscious in your children's lives is most important. I find a lot of mums need a few wines every night! I even know women who don't socialise with me because I don't drink wine every day."

"I speak to so many mums that have gone opposite to me, they never used to drink but now find it easy to consume a bottle a night. It really seems to coincide with stress a lot. I hate that I wasted my youth drinking so much but love that it isn't a priority anymore. I was really worried about myself for a long time."

"I feel like as mothers we are expected to do so much. Being the primary carer for our child, the touch stone for our families, work, don't work, groceries, household organisation and chores, it's all so much and that's not even half of it. We are expected to be sober and responsible whilst fathers are fine to have afternoon beers or evenings with friends at the pub and yet, so many memes and social media posts talk about the consumption of wine as a coping mechanism. Mothers degrade and judge each other for their opinions on drinking or not drinking because it makes them feel better when society and social media and situations promote both sides of the same coin. It's so confusing."

"Drinking alcohol after a bad day with the kids NEVER made me feel genuinely better."

"I was just sitting at home have a glass of wine thinking I wish I didn't need it (and I am sure I don't), when I saw this email! I had to do the survey!"

"A lot of my mum friends seem to drink a lot & are quite vocal about NEEDING to drink because they are stressed & having a glass of wine or more helps them relax. Personally, I think drinking only makes them more stressed especially if they wake up each morning with a hangover. It must be difficult to juggle all that we do as mums whilst nursing a sore head & feeling like crap. Feeling like this each day would make me feel stressed too & I don't think I could be the best version of myself for my kids either."

"I find that when I go out to dinner with other mums, they tend to have a few drinks because they can 'let their hair down' without the kids around. Don't know if that helps but when they are out, they will tend to drink more than when around their kids. Don't think they drink because of being mums though."

"I really don't feel the need to 'have a bottle of wine' after a hard day of parenting. I never have. But as one mother kindly informed me (after she told me she has a drinking problem) I have a cake problem. Perhaps your survey should include any vices? I probably soothe my hard parenting days by food calories and not alcohol. Great survey."

"It's a bad habit that can sneak up on you. It shouldn't be advertised as a joke on social media and I don't like friends posts of drinking alcohol. To me, it's no different to any other drug or addictive substance. It affects so many families negatively, yet we are so desensitised and accepting."

"I think that as long as a mother is able to care for the child or there is a responsible adult to do that (dad, grandparents, aunt, uncle etc) then a mum should be able to drink as much as she likes. The only time it becomes an issue is if it is putting the children in danger/neglect or the drinking becomes a problem."

"Thank you for sharing that you gave up drinking. A few years ago, a FB friend started sharing articles and her opinion about the idea that mums drink a lot of wine. I am working on becoming more self-aware and mindful. Your sharing is helping me to look at myself. I'm not ready to give up drinking yet but knowing that you have makes me a little less afraid to."

"I'm finding it hard to cut down. I want to. But I get home from work and I'm responsible for all the tedious mother things. By the time I sit down I just want to relax and feel human again. Wine helps me do that. I've put on too much weight as my consumption has increased recently. I NEED to break this habit."

"I think mothers drink more than people realise, and most are developing drinking problems. I am concerned about more than a few mums drinking."

"I feel strongly that, as with other choices women make, we should not be judged for how much we drink provided that it does not impact on the care of any children or the health of the mum in any major way. I am so aware of the stereotype of drinking mums but honestly just laugh it off. I do think that being judgemental about the amount of alcohol consumed might force those women who are using it as a crutch (i.e. more than they should or is healthy) to stay hidden and not come forward looking for help and support. It's not as big an issue as teenage underage binge drinking which is far more harmful because it's seen as 'cool'. By your forties, most women I know don't seek that kind of social reinforcement. I think most (with the exception of those who really have a problem) are able to make the decision to have a drink based on better thought patterns."

"Thanks for doing this! I haven't thought about my alcohol intake and honesty although I ticked that I'm happy with the amount of alcohol that I drink I feel like maybe I can be more conscious of my alcohol intake."

"Being a mother is the hardest job I've ever had. I definitely used to use alcohol as a crutch to help cope. It got to the point where I couldn't cope without a drink. It took me years to get to a point of accepting that reality and making the tough decision to give up altogether. I hope to be able to drink in moderation again one day in the future.

Thank you for doing this study, I think this is a really important topic x."

"Thanks for doing this work and I'm so inspired by your posts! I do think mums need to be more supportive of non-drinkers. During times when I have reduced to zero alcohol, I feel like there is a lot of pressure to 'have fun' or join in."

"I think alcohol can easily creep up to become a habit, and once it's a habit does that mean you're addicted? I could very easily drink daily because I enjoy a drink and have done so in the past (whilst being a Mum and before being a mum). Stress, monotony and boredom of being at home with tantrum-throwing, messy kids with a perpetual sink full of dirty dishes can just make you feel like a glass of wine too. It's not all about social pressure and media advertising. I can quite happily knock back a few glasses at home on my own, or with other adults. This year I stopped drinking all together for the first four months, and now stick to weekends. I'm happy with that. I don't want long-term consequences to my health from drinking too much too frequently."

"Mothers can't win. You drink, you don't drink. You drink, then it depends on what kind of alcohol you're drinking. What can you do?"

Survey Summary

When I first had the idea for the survey, it came out of a genuine interest to see if others felt as I did. I wondered if my feelings and opinions would be supported or rebuked and there was a healthy dose of each side, I feel.

Although there were some common reasons these

mothers drink or not, the results show me that their personal experiences, reasons and opinions are just that—personal to them, their beliefs and their circumstances.

You will take from the results what you will—worry or relief, justification or concern. I hope it's helped to make us a little more mindful.

STRATEGIES FOR SOBRIETY

By now you know why I quit, how I did it and the awesome things have happened since I did.

I want to share with you some things that helped me to stay sober and are continuing to help. Because, let's be real, this is still a recent change.

Also, it would be remiss of me to not give a balanced picture of the not-so-positive changes that have happened since I quit alcohol. So let's get these out of the way before we move on to taking action.

There are two main things that I've lost since quitting.

The magical ability to instantly relax

Even turning the cap of a full bottle of wine was enough to send a trigger to my brain that sent my body into instant relaxation.

Wine was coming, as was the 'blur'. It would be ok.

While I know it was a temporary fix to my problems, I miss that feeling and haven't found a replacement yet. That said, meditation helps me switch off.

The easy small talk

It isn't that I miss these types of conversations, but it's a conversation I can no longer be a part of. And now I'm so hyper-alert to the fact that the talk about alcohol is so prevalent, especially online, which is the professional world I live in.

It might be sharing wine-themed memes on social media or spending hours talking about what wine pairs beautifully with what or recounting drunken memories and events. The only thing I can add to those conversations now is my regret. And that wouldn't go down too well with wine-loving friends and peers.

So, rather than be Debbie downer, I steer clear of alcohol chat as much as possible and if the conversation heads that way, I'll bring it back to something else or excuse myself.

All that's lost isn't missed though and I'm happy to have relinquished the fear, anxiety and guilt that ate me up every day. Add to that list the future fuckups that would have inevitably happened as I drank more and more.

Following my experience, here are some of my strategies for cutting down on alcohol or cutting it out altogether.

Set a date

Whether you're going sober or looking to reduce the amount you drink, I think there needs to be a day and time where that new life and new mindset begins.

For me, it was the day before I finished reading, "How to Stop Drinking for Women".

As I took that final sip of wine, I knew it was the last one for me. Everything about it from the taste to how it made me feel screamed it was the last one.

For you, perhaps you decide right here, right now, you no longer drink. Or you no longer drink on weekdays. Or you no longer drink more than a certain amount.

Or it might help to set a date soon where you know that when you reach that date, everything changes. That isn't to say you go hell for leather in the run up to it. But you either carry on as you are or slowly reduce your alcohol intact so when that date arrives, you're not going cold turkey if that doesn't suit you.

Get support

Support is essential for staying on track with most major life decisions and might come in the form of family, friends, mentors, books, articles, groups, forums or more. Or a combination of many of these things.

What helped me was talking publicly about my decision as it attracted other mums who wanted to do the same thing. We became a little community that shared why we were making changes, how we were doing it and offered each other encouragement along the way.

I also have loved reading other people's stories and journeys about going alcohol-free. It helps me to not only get tips from them but also to remind myself I'm not alone. There's a huge movement now of women cutting down on or cutting out alcohol for similar reasons to my own.

You can also check out my Resources section at the end of this book for the actual resources I used when quitting and ever since.

Give the problem a name

This is where it gets controversial. According to Carr, all

alcohol consumers are addicted to the drug but at a different stage. Having read the book, I get this.

That isn't to say I tar every alcoholic drinker with the 'you're a big ole addict' brush and I'm not condemning anyone for their own choices.

However, it helped me to realise my relationship with alcohol was that it was an addiction. It gave what I deemed my lack of control, a condition. And it was a condition that had a possible cure and I could therefore start the steps to healing the condition and overcoming the addiction.

This mindset may totally resonate with you too. Or it may not. I found the realisation I had an addiction, not just a habit, liberating.

Revisit your 'why'

Why do you want to cut back or cut out alcohol?

For me, it was the realisation the solution I thought it was giving me was in fact a lie. Drinking to excess was worsening my problems.

Allen Carr Clinics believes drinking alcohol:

"Doesn't provide any genuine benefits or advantages whatsoever. Drinkers are simply relieving the physical withdrawal created by the previous drink. Everything else is smoke and mirrors, illusions created by our misinterpretation of the process."

This was gold for me but it's also an ongoing challenge and a fact I need to keep coming back to regularly.

Carr's book helped me to see whilst I might get a very

short-term fix from the effects of alcohol, they soon wore off unless I continued to drink more and more. And then having continued to drink, and to excess, my original problems that led me to drink worsened over time.

I'll share an example, to put this into perspective:

One reason I drank was to 'relax' after a hard day or long week. I felt I needed something that instantly made me shut off from the busy-ness and the stress and move me into 'weekend mode' or 'evening mode'. I wanted to switch my mind off to the hard things that might have happened that day, or even the good things that were still overwhelming me because I was so busy.

And it worked. From turning the cap of a bottle of wine to finishing the last glass from it, the rest of the day faded away and I could happily exist in my bubble of relaxation. Or what I thought was so.

I would inevitably go to bed feeling like a failure for drinking again. And then wake up feeling tired and drained after a restless night and face the reality of my busy life with even less energy, creativity and drive.

Any challenges I had didn't go away. They were masked or put 'on hold' but they were still there waiting for me in the stone-cold sober light of day.

Whether I was drinking to relax, to feel more confident, to block out my fears or all the many other excuses I told myself, it was nothing more than a temporary fix. A break from reality. And when the alcohol wore off, the issues remained, only I was in an even less powerful state to deal with them than before I'd taken the first drink.

I continue to go back to the reasons I quit often, and sometimes multiple times a week. Be very clear about why you are making this change, understand the benefits that will come and be resolute to stick to it by revisiting your 'why' regularly.

Enjoy the freedom

I still pinch myself throughout the day when I realise I'm no longer battling an alcohol addiction of any kind.

In fact, removing the choice of alcohol from my life means I can focus my attention more on options that enhance my life instead.

I'm no longer tied to choices, events, venues and decisions where alcohol plays a factor in my life. I can go anywhere, do anything and make decisions with a clear and focused mind.

My new clarity and drive might have closed off some sensations, conversations and experiences but it's opened so much more to me. I didn't realise life after alcohol would be liberating.

I'll share some practical steps I put into place after I stopped drinking:

Alternative drinks

Another challenge was what to pour into my booze-free cup. Because that cup is now so glaringly dry.

I tried all sorts: water, juicing, smoothies, kombucha, relaxation drinks, tea and more. I've enjoyed the variety and the hit on my bank balance has been way less than the wine.

Replacing alcohol isn't as simple as switching it for a healthier drink because it all depends on your reason for drinking in the first place.

For those of us who drink to relax, a glass of chilled water isn't going to have the same effect, right?

For the mums who are downing a gin and tonic because they think it will give them the courage to network at a business event, removing the gin might not do the trick.

Then, for the mother who drinks a bottle of wine each night to blur out the stress, the tension, the mundane or the anxiety, will any alcohol-free drink give them that same buzz? Unlikely.

So, whilst there are many healthier drink options to choose from, if you're looking for an alternative to alcohol, you need to think about *why* you were drinking alcohol in the first place.

What is the real need you need to address?

Why does drinking alcohol feel so good?

Oxford Dictionaries defines alcohol as:

"A colourless volatile flammable liquid which is produced by the natural fermentation of sugars and is the intoxicating constituent of wine, beer, spirits, and other drinks, and is also used as an industrial solvent and as fuel."

Nice.

Otherwise known as ethanol, it makes you feel drunk.

Healthline says:

"Alcohol is one of the most popular psychoactive substances in the world. It can have powerful effects on your mood and mental state. By reducing self-consciousness and shyness, alcohol may encourage people to act without inhibition. At the same time, it impairs judgement and promotes behaviour people may end up regretting."

It got me thinking about the things I could do to replace alcohol with a healthier alternative or substitute. Not just by replacing the substance itself, but the time I was spending thinking about drinking and the actual time drinking.

Whether you're cutting out alcohol altogether, or cutting back, be curious to trying more new things. Let's call it your Non-Booze Bucket List.

Here are some drinks and activities to do instead of drinking alcohol:

- Water – still and sparkling
- Juice
- Smoothies
- Tea
- Coffee
- Relaxation drinks
- Alcohol-free beverages

A note on the latter. Allen Carr Clinics advises against alcohol-free beverages for this reason:

"Avoid any form of substitution, be it excessive food, soft drinks or alcohol-free imitations of alcoholic drinks. By using a substitute you're perpetuating the illusion you're missing out on something – drinking does nothing for you, there is no void to fill."

I've tried a few alcohol-removed wines and beers and they haven't caused me to relapse or affect my resolve about not drinking. However, I asked a few sober peers about their experience and for some, it's off the table altogether as it reminds them too much of the real thing and trigger their cravings.

Alternative activities

- Have an early night
- Read a book – to yourself or the kids
- Write a book
- Start a blog
- Watch a movie
- Work out
- Plan your budget
- Plan a holiday
- Have a bath or shower
- Wash your hair
- Play outside with the kids
- Manicure or pedicure
- Make a batch of freezer meals
- Tidy/declutter a room
- Clean
- Home décor project
- Learn to play an instrument
- Play a board game
- Play a smartphone game
- Play solitaire
- Draw pictures
- Scroll social media
- Call a friend
- Write a letter
- Read and reply to emails
- Declutter email folders
- Have sex
- Kiss your partner
- Get a massage
- Give a massage
- Arrange flowers (nah, seriously)
- Braid your child's hair

- Listen to music
- Create a playlist
- Watch YouTube videos
- Spend time in nature
- Take selfies
- Update photos in frames

What can you add to the list?

I'm a constant rotation of many on the list although you're unlikely to walk into my home and find me arranging daisies any time soon but I'm catering for all tastes peeps!

I reached out to some friends who don't drink to learn more about what motivates them to either cut back on alcohol or avoid it altogether.

Nicole said:

"I was a heavy social drinker before I fell pregnant with my first baby and over the following six years, I was either pregnant or breastfeeding. I was so excited to be able to drink again but quickly realised how awful it made me feel. Not to mention it didn't even taste good. In the end, I decided it wasn't worth it. If I'd managed to have a social life without alcohol for the past six years, then I'd be just fine without it!"

I love learning from some of my celebrity idols too. In her article "What Being Sober Has Meant to Me", Brené Brown talks about attending her first Alcoholics Anonymous meeting and quitting alcohol and cigarettes:

"At first I struggled to feel 'drunk enough' to belong at AA."

She goes on to say:

"I've only really missed drinking three or four times –

mostly when I need a way to medicate overwhelming anxiety. As much as I try to work a "live and let live" vibe, I've watched "civilised drinking" ravage the lives of so many families and friends that I've developed no interest in it at all."

Brené attended AA meetings during her first year of sobriety and still works the program.

My friend Eva said:

"The first month was the hardest for me and so to combat any cravings I found it helpful to have a sparkling mineral water with a wedge of lime. Not only did this give me something tasty and healthy to drink, the fact that I had something in my hand filled the space where my wine glass used to be.

When I did drink, I had a bad habit of drinking when I was hungry because the effects of the alcohol were quicker. After stopping alcohol, particularly in the first month, I always made sure I'd had something to eat so my hunger cravings didn't turn into a craving for wine."

Karen, mum of two, wanted to cut back on her alcohol intake, but not quit completely. She shared how she did this:

"I did a few things to cut back on drinking wine. First, I stopped buying wine. As there was none in the house, it meant I had to make a big effort to go out to buy some. When it was in the fridge, it was all too easy to open a bottle. And the second thing that helped was when I was craving a glass, I had a big drink of something else instead. (Water or coffee.)

I found that often I was fancying a glass of wine because I was thirsty. Finally, I often have a drink with dinner in my favourite crystal wine glasses! It's usually water or sparkling water but it feels like I'm enjoying a nice drink with my meal that way!"

Being around friends who drink alcohol

As you know, I decided up front to tell everyone in my life that I'd kicked alcohol. I did so partly to gain their support too. It helped they knew not just that I'd quit but the reasons why and they've never sought to tempt me off the wagon I hauled myself upon.

Maybe it's an age thing. But as much as my circle of friends like a drink, our big boozy bender days are pretty much a thing of the past, so I haven't needed to avoid any friends particularly.

Of course, there are some friends I had nothing in common with except for bonding over wine and I've moved myself away from that over the years anyway. By bonding, I don't mean in the good positive sense.

I mean those conversations where, after a few drinks, you put the world to rights in a negative and miserable way, often resulting in bitching, whining and hurtfulness. I don't need that.

As Rachel Hollis says in "Girl, Wash Your Face!":

"You become who you surround yourself with" and I don't want to be like those people.

I don't feel the need to surround myself with sober women only either, just those who support my decisions without judgement. I can happily spend time with other people who are drinking a little.

Nicole has this advice about going out with friends who drink:

"When I am out at social gatherings, I like to make or

order sparkling water or soft drinks but add garnishes like lemon or a sprig of mint. It makes it look like you're drinking alcohol, so you avoid the "Are you pregnant?" questions and also just feels a bit more fun and inclusive rather than a regular drink."

Alcohol and the workplace

Given I work from home, I'm lucky to no longer have the temptation of after-work drinks. Or the cart that's wheeled around the office at 3.30pm on a Friday afternoon to signal work is out and wine is in.

Does your workplace have that too? It could be an Australian thing and it was an event I thought rocked in my corporate years.

These days, it's work conferences, meet ups and brand events where the temptation to drink looms.

If you spend five minutes on social media, as a blogger, you'll be inundated with social posts from friends, pages and groups pushing wine-fuelled events where you can 'let your hair down', 'meet other mums in business' and 'network'.

And I'm all for those events. I love to network. The world of self-employment can be so isolating, and these events are a vital opportunity to reconnect with other like-minded women who are going through the same juggles and struggles as me.

So far, I haven't been tempted to drink wine, and since proclaiming to the world I was an alcohol-free zone, no one has even offered me a glass. So that's easy.

But what about you? If you work in a job or industry where there is pressure to drink when you'd rather not, I say stand tall and hold your ground.

You might not want to be as vocal as me of course, but don't feel shame in telling people you would rather not drink, or you're happy with a small amount.

Of course, there'll always be the idiots who assume you're pregnant and obnoxiously shout that out for all to hear. *Aren't those people annoying?*

Think of some ways to steer the conversations you're having away from alcohol and if you're asked why you're not drinking, you have three choices.

You either tell them it's none of their business, you tell them the true reasons why (whatever they might be for you) or you go the route of lying.

E.g. "I'm on antibiotics" or "I'm driving", etc.

Of course, you *could* be on medication or driving home from the event, so you needn't lie at all.

But find a strategy that works for you that results in the least stress for you too. Only you choose what you put in your body and you're not obliged to answer to anyone about that.

Nights out and events

As well as work events, there are general nights out, birthdays, weddings and more to look forward to doing sober.

There'll likely be the same nosy questions from some about why you're not drinking or drinking less.

For me, it came back to informing people proudly that I don't drink and then moving the conversation swiftly along to subjects not related to alcohol.

If you're heading out on a night out or to an event, have a plan.

Decide in advance what you're going to drink and even eat. Knowing before you arrive what your plan is will give you confidence and when you're asked what you want to drink, you already have some go-to responses.

If you're the one organising an event, consider establishments and venues that don't even serve alcohol but, unless you don't want to go out, don't stay in. What I mean is, don't feel you need to avoid social occasions because you're drinking less or going sober.

For me, it helped to continue as normal, to eat and drink in the same places with the same people. I didn't ask any of my friends to stop drinking but many now choose not to drink when they're with me. They tell me it's an opportunity for them to have a 'night off' from wine and I'm more than happy to be their excuse for that.

Do what works for you to reduce temptation and stay on track.

The Sex

Yes, I went there. And this won't be relevant for all women but for me, alcohol and sex has always gone hand in hand.

I mean, there have been plenty of occasions when I've had sober sex of course, but often I've had at least one glass of 'Dutch courage' before stripping off and getting down.

I thought for a long time that drunk sex was better sex. I had more confidence; less body hang ups and edges became blurred.

I was more adventurous, liberated and interesting in

the bedroom.

Until I stopped drinking. Then, I'll be totally honest, all that stopped. In fact, it was about six weeks until I finally had the confidence to jump the hubs again.

How did it go? It was awkward as hell, thanks for asking.

Seriously awkward. Like that first kiss where we clashed teeth only it was under a duvet and the teeth were the least of our issues.

It was a lot more bump than grind and it took a good few bumps to find our groove that night. But we did, and after a dodgy start it was another big tick on the 'things that got better when I stopped drinking alcohol' list.

Despite the initial awkwardness, I didn't think about my body hang ups once.

And yes, it might not have been our most mind-blowing encounter. Sorry Mr M, I'll stop this sharing soon I promise! But it was good sex, I slept soundly afterwards and the next day I remembered everything we'd done and how good it felt.

That was liberating. Who knew sober sex could feel even better than wild-abandoned, drunk sex?

Every day is a Sex School day. And it got good. R*eally* good.

So, when it comes to sober sex for you, don't assume it won't be as good. Don't knock it 'til you've tried it. So they say.

WHAT'S NEXT FOR ME?

So, life after alcohol is more than fulfilling. In fact, the time spent drinking, and thinking about drinking, can be much better put to use in my humble opinion.

This mummy does not need wine.

But why-oh-why is being a mum now synonymous with drinking wine and gin?

And why is it deemed acceptable for the media, and social media, to put the "mummy needs wine" message to us on the daily?

Would "Mummy needs sugar?" or "Mummy needs cocaine?" be as acceptable.

#mummyneedswine

#mummyneedsgin

#mummywinetime

"TAG A MUM WHO BLACKED OUT AFTER WINE LAST NIGHT (LAUGHING EMOJI)"

Plus, a million and one other freely used hashtags on social media. #mommyneedswine has over 15k users on Instagram alone and #winemom has over 51k.

Pretty sure 'old me' had used those.

My friends Sara agrees:

"The modern motherhood narrative that has developed is a series of contradictions. On one hand, we should all feel #soblessed for the gift of children but on the other hand, mum life is HARD, and we all need to drink alcohol to survive it. As any mum will know, the reality is a glorious mess of highs and lows, laughter and tears. The messaging around alcohol as a part of the motherhood experience has made me feel uncomfortable, but I know in the past I have been guilty of perpetrating it. My reality is I drink less now than I did before I had kids. I don't drink so I can handle my kids and I don't drink to get drunk like I did in my twenties. If you believe the media/social media, every mum is cracking open a bottle of wine every night and drinking full oversized glasses of the stuff. It normalises it. And for people who have a healthy relationship with alcohol, they can scroll past and it won't affect them. But for others, I can 100% see how it could create a problem or exacerbate an existing problem they have."

I never thought I would give up drinking. I couldn't imagine my life without 'wine o'clock'. But you know what, #wineoclock is fucked (despite it's nearly 2 million Instagram occurrences).

The message that all mums *need* wine or gin or 'mummy's special juice' is nothing short of horrific. *Needs it? Really?*

And I bought into it. Hell, I perpetuated its promotion too. It made me believe alcohol addiction was normal.

We were all doing it, so it was ok. We all *needed* to drink to get through mum life.

Does mummy need wine?

I can tell you after ditching it, I'm mum-ing it just fine.

I wish I could have controlled my alcohol consumption but, hands up, I could not.

And if you see yourself in any of my story, you're not

alone as my survey results show.

Do I wish everyone would stop drinking alcohol?

In a way, yes. Apart from the health benefits we all know about, steering clear of the booze greatly lessens the risk of becoming addicted to it. It's better to leave the fight than risk injury.

Plus, it would remove the temptation for me, and the many other women like me, who develop an addiction.

Maybe you think the book I read brainwashed me into sobriety? Maybe I think the peer pressure you might have experienced brainwashed you into alcohol usage? Perhaps we have both thoughts sometimes? But our opinions are our own.

For me, getting drunk meant zoning out and zoning out meant I could be someone other than who I thought I was. I could forget my inadequacies and pretend to be a better version of myself: confident, happier, sexier, more fun.

Now I've quit wine, I realise I was already all of those things and if anything, the alcohol trap took away my self-awareness and made me hide my true self.

For example, I'm quite the sex pot already, thanks very much. I might be tone deaf with no rhythm but I'm confident enough to get up there and sing and dance anyway.

And with my rediscovered confidence I realise I have also regained my perception. I listen more and rant less. I might be the loudest talker in the group but I'm less likely to say something offensive or obnoxious.

Nothing good has changed for the worst. I'm no longer in mourning for the life I had because it's still there, just better.

I no longer need alcohol to issue me with a permission slip to be the person I want to be. I'm already her.

The wine has gone but the family, friends and fun remains.

Minus the hangover, hit to my bank balance and self-esteem.

If my story has resonated with you, you might consider quitting alcohol yourself now.

Whilst I've shown you how I did it, I understand the road to sobriety might not be as easy for everyone. Later, I will share the resources I have used to get and stay sober.

SUMMARY

If someone had told me in the past, I would write a book about how I became addicted to alcohol, I wouldn't have believed them for a moment.

And if they'd said I would eventually be sober, I would have laughed in their face.

Having prided myself for years on my ability to stay in control, even in the face of extreme adversity, alcohol addiction was not going to be any part of my life's story.

Until the day it was.

Sharing how that happened, how I recognised the problem and the steps I took to overcome it has been a cathartic experience for me. And I hope will help other women who might be in the same boat, or about to set sail.

My newfound sobriety is just that—new. But in this chapter of my life, it's working for me and I intend to be here for longer, continuing to create and share new chapters in the book of my life.

The new 'me' is a stronger and more self-aware version of myself than I could have imagined, and I like myself now a lot more than I did in my drinking days.

I am present, reliable, focused, resilient and oh-so-much happier now. In the words of Disney's Elsa, "I'm free".

I've let go of the alcohol trap and I am now dealing with my shit. Not solving it all but dealing with it. Not drinking it away.

I also know my confidence to quit has inspired others. Sara told me recently:

"At the time you made the decision, I didn't really get it, but as you've unpacked the impact alcohol was having in your life, and I can see the difference it has made to you, it's been great. It seems like it truly was the right decision for you."

And it wasn't 'being a mum' that specifically led me to alcohol. Or any particular areas of motherhood that turned drinking too much into an addiction.

It was all of it.

The accumulation of busy mum life, wife life, work life, stressful incidents and health issues that had me reach my limit.

Pressing the 'Pause' button wasn't an option and there was no holiday from having to hold it all together because I had a family who depended on me.

My two babies, my husband, they'd fought cancer with me, and they needed me to keep being here.

I hadn't realised the extent being diagnosed with cancer so early in motherhood had affected me. I was spiralling inside when everyone around me needed me to thrive and told me I should be.

Society places a pressure on mothers to be perfect and for cancer survivors to be eternally grateful.

And I am so bloody grateful. But I'm also still in shock, still reeling and still pulling myself together.

Alcohol was my crutch; my time out. My alternate universe where life was good and easy and somewhat blurry. Blurry was comforting.

It took quitting alcohol and peeling off the wine bottle shaped bandage to see how much I'd been ignoring myself.

Heartache, isolation, cancer, anxiety. I was self-medicating away all of that hurt with alcohol.

Whilst writing this book, I've had many moments where I've questioned if sharing my story is the right decision.

My darkest secrets have the potential to embarrass my family, and me, for life.

But this is me, face-down in the arena that Brené encourages us to charge into. As she so wisely said:

"We can choose courage, or we can choose comfort, but we can't have both, not at the same time."

So, I'm feeling brave and daring by sharing.

Then, out of nowhere, and email appeared in my Inbox from Renée after following my journey through sobriety on my blog and social media:

"I don't know if you know just how much you've inspired me to get sober (and more important, to stay sober)! Our stories are so similar, and every time you've posted an update on social media about your sobriety over these last few months, I've thought to myself 'I want what she's got!'"

And it's clear to me now I'm not only sharing my story cathartically anymore. Some other mums are crying out for this alcohol-free movement too and they're grateful I'm putting my experience out there.

I put my embarrassment aside because as Brené said:

"When you judge yourself for needing help, you judge those you are helping."

So, do we all need to quit booze?

I'm not of the mindset all alcohol is the Devil's work and I'm not advocating for everyone to stop drinking.

Right now, even one glass is entirely off the cards for me and I can't see it ever being a possibility. At least not a sensible one. It's too soon and I'm still too addicted to a substance I believe did nothing good for me.

Quitting alcohol has given me back so much of the control I've lost, from heartbreaks to cancer.

These days, going out and getting wasted isn't on my agenda. I have two small kids, a husband, a busy life and lots of laundry. I don't have the time or funds to waste on alcohol.

The issue was the habit. A bad habit that turned into an addiction.

I hope I always feel like my life is better without alcohol. And I hope the mourning for not drinking anymore continues to fade away.

It's the end of a toxic relationship. Alcohol wasn't good for me and it wasn't contributing anything positive to my life. Instead, it was preventing me from being my best self. My real self.

I never want to fall back into the alcohol trap again. I value my freedom too much for that.

In the early months of quitting, I longed to be one of those people who was happy to drink the occasional glass of wine every few weeks or on special occasions. Or only one night per week. And I've been that person before, only not for very long.

I've never been a 'one glass' girl and I doubt I ever would be. Whilst I believe we can correct many bad habits, why would I waste time and effort into making myself *less* dependent on alcohol yet dependent all the same?

Alcohol did nothing good for me and I haven't lost a thing by quitting.

What I have gained is time. I'm hopeful my improved health will lead to me being around for my family for more years to come.

I'm no longer tied to licensed venues and wine lists and the time I invest into my family and friends is quality time.

My evenings are calm, less frantic, peaceful and productive. I no longer struggle to focus or waste my mornings shaking off the dustiness of the night before.

At work I'm clear-headed, creative and empower myself to reach my goals.

I'm mindful of being present in my family's life and in my own. I'm grateful, happy and free.

I have more time for the people and the things that matter in my life now. I have more time for me and to be me.

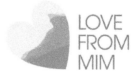

LOVE
FROM
MIM

RESOURCES

Here are some of the books, apps and resources that helped me stay on track:

- "How to Stop Drinking for Women" by Allen Carr
- "The Unexpected Benefits of Being Sober" by Catherine Gray
- "Rising Strong" by Brené Brown
- "Atomic Habits" by James Clear
- "I Am Sober" Phone app
- Cancer Council NSW: https://www.cancercouncil.com.au/
- Drinkaware website: https://www.drinkaware.co.uk/
- My Blog
- www.lovefrommim.com
- My Facebook Group:
- https://www.facebook.com/groups/424225781697647/

I love to follow hashtags on Instagram to find like-minded people, such as:

- #soberaf
- #sobermums
- #sobermoms
- #soberwomen

You can read the full results of my 2019 survey into Motherhood and Alcohol here:

https://lovefrommim.com/motherhood-alcohol-2019-survey-results/

Here are a few uplifting quotes from my favourite authors and coaches that always keep me motivated and on track:

- Brené Brown: "We are the authors of our own lives. We write our own daring endings."
- Kris Carr: "Simple steps lead to profound change."
- Rachel Hollis: "Only you have the power to change your own life."
- Brené Brown: "I realised that my sobriety is not a limitation. Sobriety isn't even a "have to" – it's a superpower."
- Jim Fortin: "Everything is 100% possible, 100% of the time".

ACKNOWLEDGEMENTS

An extra special thanks to my husband, my children and my parents for their everlasting love and support. You are my everything, my purpose, my whole life.

To my girl band (and you know who you are) for having faith in me, encouraging me and taking me seriously when I said I was quitting something else. I actually did it this time!

To Karen McDermott, Lisa Burling, Renee Conoulty, Dannielle Line and Lisa Wolstenholme for guiding and helping me to make an actual, real life book. Thank you for your amazing expertise and patience. Let this be the first of many?

I would also like to thank my beautiful online community of readers, followers and coaches who allowed me to share the ups and downs of my life with them over the past five years. Thank you for your words and messages of love and support as well as your continual kindness and faith in me. You mean the world to me.

Love from Mim x x x

ABOUT THE AUTHOR

Mim Jenkinson is a British, married mother of two and lives with her family in Australia.

A professional storyteller, Mim runs her own blog as well as providing content strategy and copywriting services to a wealth of clients. She especially enjoys writing for an audience of women and her work has appeared on the Huffington Post, Thrive Global, Kidspot, Essential Baby and Tell Me Baby.

Away from the keyboard, Mim is an avid fan of country music, pretty stationery and Outlander.

Find out more about Mim at www.lovefrommim.com and on social media @lovefrommim